CULTURE, POLITICS, AND MEDICINE IN COSTA RICA

CULTURE, POLITICS, AND MEDICINE IN COSTA RICA

An Anthropological Study of Medical Change

Setha M. Low

ISBN 0-913178-01-2

Printed in the United States of America
91 90 89 88 87 86 85 6 5 4 3 2 1

TO

THE PEOPLE OF COSTA RICA

CONTENTS

ILLUSTRATIONS

TABLES

ACKNOWLEDGMENTS

This research would not have been possible without the cooperation and support of many people to whom I remain indebted. I would like to thank Dr. Guido Miranda G. of the Caja Costarricense de Seguro Social; Dr. Carlos Saenz, Dr. Guido Jimenez, Dr. Gallegos Chacon, and Dr. Mora Aquilar of Hospital Calderon Guardia; Dr. Sanchez-Bourbon of Hospital Mexico; Dr. José Manuel Quirce, Dr. Pacheco Cartin and Lic. Roberto Loria of Hospital San Juan de Dios; Dr. Alvarenga and Dr. Pacheco of Hospital Psiquiátrico Manuel Antonio Chapui; Dr. Oscar Alfaro R., Dr. A. Alfaro Sotela and Dra. Virginia Barquero of the Ministerio de Salud; and Dr. Rodrigo Gutierrez of the Escuela de Medicina, Universidad de Costa Rica for their assistance in the study of the medical care system. These dedicated doctors and administrators generously contributed their time, publications, knowledge and guidance to my research and ideas. I especially would like to express my gratitude to those doctors and patients of the general medicine and psychiatric sections who allowed me to interview them and observe their medical consultations although their names are not included to protect the confidentiality of both the doctor-patient and researcher-informant relationships.

Special thanks are extended to my research assistant Bruce Newman who collected the 117 before-and-after interviews and accompanied me during the family interviews and to Norma Jimènez Volio who collected detailed observations of pharmacy patrons and clients.

While in the field I was fortunate to know Professors Gonzalo Adis Castro, Janina Bonilla de Ulloa, María Eugenia Bozzoli de Wille, José Antonio Camacho, María Eugenia López de Piza, William Reuben, Samuel Z. Stone and Lillian Stover of the Universidad de Costa Rica who provided support, discussion and valuable advice. Visiting anthropologists George Foster, Dwight B. Heath, Marshall T. Newman, Lucile F. Newman and Miles Richardson added a much needed perspective through their experienced suggestions and comments. Upon my return, Renée Fox, Francis E. Johnston, Ian McHarg, Lucile Newman, and Nathan Sivin encouraged me to complete this book. I am grateful to my colleagues for their scholarly concern and friendship.

My thanks also go to typists Martha Kroch and Kay Mower, copyeditors Linda Rachele Burke and Lydia Greiner, and to the following journals and their editors for permission to reprint material related to the present study: *Medical Anthropology* (Robert C.

Ness, editor), *Milbank Memorial Fund Quarterly/Health and Society* (David Willis, editor), *Social Science and Medicine* (Charles Leslie, editor), *Urban Anthropology* (Jack Rollwagen, editor). A careful reading of the manuscript by Arthur Kleinman, Martin Meyerson and Lucile Newman improved its style and content, however its final form and conclusions are solely those of the author.

The research data were collected over a period of twenty-one months from October 1972 through August 1974 supported by a National Institute of Mental Health Combination Research Fellowship, and during the summers of 1976 and 1979 with the support of the University of Pennsylvania. Supplemental funds were provided by a Special Career Fellowship in the Social Sciences and Humanities and a Center for Latin American Studies Fellowship from the University of California, Berkeley. The writing of this book completed with the support and encouragement of Michael S. Batcher, Myra Bluebond-Langner, Erve Chambers, and Denise O'Brien.

FOREWORD

Scientific medicine has become a symbol of modernization with increased life expectancy, decreased infant mortality, control of public health aspects of community living as internationally accepted indices of success.

This extraordinary book provides a case analysis of Costa Rica; a modernizing nation engaging in a serious effort at democratization of medical care as a key priority of government policy. It raises a number of questions. In a society where health appears to be a national obsession, can health services keep up with demand? Can government support and control of health care escape bureaucratization? How do families respond to this health policy? These questions and others are addressed in a multilevel study using the integrated methods of medical anthropology.

Medical Anthropology, as a field, emphasizes interactive processes, both sides of the story. Building an integrated approach to these transactions, Dr. Low moves from institutional to personal acknowledgment of the special role of health as a measure of well-being in the Costa Rican setting and of the transcending quality of the communications between patient and doctor.

It is indeed an Anthropological Study of Culture Change. The integration of methods of observation, interviews with administrators, physicians and patients, and intensive family interviews provide a rare opportunity to view both the focal institutions and where they fit into the lives of people not immediately engaged with the system. The success of a medical system beyond the numbers of life expectancy concerns the interactions between a practitioner and a help-seeking person and the degree to which this interaction is helpful to the patient and validating to the medical system. One of the most telling of Dr. Low's observations is that "the patients who use a variety of health care solutions tend to be the most satisfied with the therapeutic outcome" (p. 105). Multiple solutions enable strategic health promoting actions involving a range of resort from indigenous herbal remedies to reliance on the intercession of folk saints. The state system of scientific medicine, however, opposes folk and supernatural forms of healing. Dr. Low has provided the field with a close study of modernization and an increasingly depersonalized structure in tension with the individual desire to maintain aspects of traditional culture and a sense of personal control in their lives.

Lucile Newman
Brown University
Providence, Rhode Island

INTRODUCTION

Culture, Politics, and Medicine examines the Costa Rican patient within the context of a developing nation's health care system. It analyzes the determinants by which the cultural and political development of the health care system affect therapeutic success and patient satisfaction. A medical anthropological approach to health care contrasts underlying cultural and family values, which influence the health behavior of the individual, with the sociopolitical structure of the medical institution, the determining factor in both the doctor-patient interaction and the course of medical treatment. The integration of historical, cultural, and political data generates a model of patient health behavior. The health behavior model suggests policy recommendations for the delivery of health care services in any medical system which has a specific ideological or political affiliation.

The study was begun with the intention of demonstrating how family and cultural values determine health behavior regardless of the institutional or professional setting. All sectors of health care, including folk medicine and popular remedies, as well as all major hospitals and clinics, were observed in order to gather information on how values and behavior were linked. In the process of this investigation, however, new hypotheses of health behavior based on the nationalization of the medical institutional structure and on political ideology emerged from the data. Thus, the study presents the important dimensions of institutional politics and cultural expectations in the determination of patient health behavior for students and practitioners in the social sciences, public health, Latin American studies, health care, and health planning. Although family values, cultural beliefs, and practices play a role in health seeking behavior, the institutional and ideological elements of a national health care system influence the quality of both doctor-patient interaction and patient satisfaction. The medical relationship is ultimately damaged and therapeutic effectiveness is impeded.

This investigation presents a model for health behavior in developing countries from the evaluation of the Costa Rican patient experience in an urban health care system. The research focus is a comparison of patient satisfaction with medical consultation within two Costa Rican medical institutions of contrasting sociopolitical history and organization. The research presents a detailed analysis of patient satisfaction in the medical setting as it illustrates the relative impact of the individual, familial, institutional, and cultural processes on health behavior and medical care.

Traditionally, Costa Rica was a society of equally poor and hardworking small landowners. The equality of social relations first shifted with the advent of coffee production; land was amassed by a few wealthy landowners who controlled coffee processing, and a growing class of landless peasant laborers evolved. Social relations changed with the increasing class inequality and a predominence of *patron-peon* (Foster 1962) relationships began to characterize transactions between these two groups. Social institutions that developed during this period, including medical hospitals and clinics, were based on the noblesse oblige concept of the provision of care by the elite to a needy peasant population. The political ideology of the charity and later public hospitals was consistent with the social reality and structure of doctor-patient relations according to the dominant elite and subordinate peasant pattern.

A second change in Costa Rican social relations and political ideology followed a period of labor unrest and the development of the first labor unions in the banana-producing zones of the republic. Through the increased participation of workers in the political process, a small minority of Communists were voted into the Legislative Assembly. A temporary political alliance in the legislative process among the members of the ruling elite, the Catholic Church, and the Communist Party produced a series of Labor and Social Security laws, which provided for worker health and disability through the creation of a new medical institution. The Social Security hospitals were infused with an egalitarian political ideology which influenced both the recruitment and performance of doctors and patients. The Costa Rican social reality had remained the same, yet the Social Security institutional structure fostered ideals of social equality and democratic process. The resulting conflict between the actual status difference of doctor and patient, and the ideologically expected social equality in role performance has negatively influenced the course of doctor-patient interaction in the Social Security setting.

Costa Rica is becoming an increasingly medicalized health culture and has adopted a nationalized health care system which limits the individual's traditional health care choices. The Social Security institution, where the conflicting expectations and realities of the doctor-patient interaction are most apparent, is mandated to take over Costa Rican hospitals and clinics by 1984. The pattern of ineffectual medical consultation, therefore, could become the norm and characterize all medical interaction. Further, the plural medical system of San José, made up of folk, popular, and professional sectors, increasingly is the target for legislation restricting paramedical practitioners and transferring indigenous methods of health care to medical institutions.

In order to document the determinants of change in Costa Rican health behavior, a description of Costa Rican health culture, the health care system, health seeking process, familial, and institutional settings is presented. The research data and analyses are integrated by the proposed health behavior model and discussed in relation to the health policy implications of the research. An overview of the research methodology can be found in the Appendix.

CHAPTER I

COSTA RICAN HEALTH CULTURE

Costa Rica: the Cultural Context

Costa Rican society, both structurally and conceptually, reflects a preoccupation with health. On any main street in the city center one is struck by the abundance of medical offices and related laboratories, clinics, and pharmacies. The national budget for 1973 allotted more money for health than for defense and internal security (*La República* 1973: 12); and the proportion of public expenses corresponding to the health sector, which increased from 9.0% in 1960 to 14.9% in 1972 (Bermudez Gomez 1974: 22), has continued to rise. The reserves of the semi-autonomous Caja Costarricense de Seguro Social (Social Security agency) are so large that it has become the major internal money lender to the national government and "has a budget equal to 40 percent of the government's annual operating budget" (Rosenberg 1981: 278).

In the major daily newspapers, *La Nación* and *La República*, there are lengthy articles reporting health hazards, health directives, or information on the opening of a new clinic or medical program. Costa Ricans worry more about their health than about their economic state (Richardson and Bode 1971). Health concerns dominate conversations and lifestyles.

Health to a Costa Rican is expressed as well-being (*bienestar*) or to be sound, or complete (*estar sano*). To achieve and maintain this well-being requires that one must *vivir tranquilo*, that is, live calmly, tranquilly, in balance with oneself and one's physical, social, and psychological environment. The experience of illness interrupts life's balance and begins a sequence of health seeking behaviors in which an individual attempts to bring the body, social relationships, and psychological attitude back into the culturally prescribed state of health. The cultural context of health, the social world in which patients search for cures and remedies, and the rules and meanings which direct those behaviors define Costa Rica's health culture.

Health culture in Costa Rica is made up of diverse religious, biomedical, and supernatural beliefs represented in a complex, pluralistic health care system which traditionally includes a variety of medical, paramedical, and folk practitioners. The threat of legislation which would restrict paramedical practitioners and the increasing numbers of biomedically trained physicians have reduced the numbers of practitioners of alternative methods. The resulting emphasis on a single mode of health care has also begun to affect what is considered culturally appropriate health behavior. The combination of these factors has characterized the process of Costa Rican health culture medicalization.

Medicalization is a concept employed by Ivan Illich in his book *Medical Nemesis* (1976) to critique the current tendency of Western society to define an increasing number of social problems as having medical solutions and therefore within the social control of biomedical practitioners. His concern is that the power politics of an expansion of medical expertise reduce the ability of the individual to resolve basic life challenges and encourage biomedical dependency. These ideas have been modified by subsequent commentary and research which identify a capitalist or commercial rather than a professional dependence as the basis for medicalization (Ferguson 1981). With either interpretation, the concept remains an important indicator of change in Latin American health care.

Renée Fox, who studied medicalization in the United States, suggests that this shift in social control further translates what was once considered a religious domain into a medical problem:

> One significant form that the process of medicalization has taken is the increase in the numbers and kinds of attitudes and behaviors that have come to be defined as illnesses and treatment of which is regarded as belonging within the jurisdiction of medicine and its practitioners. In an earlier, more religiously oriented era of a modern Western society like our own, some of these same kinds of attitudes and behaviors were considered sinful rather than sick, and they fell under the authorities for a different kind of diagnosis, treatment, and control. (Fox 1977: 11).

This aspect of medicalization, in which religious symbols and systems of healing are supplemented or modified by biomedical symbols, is taking the control of personal health care out of the hands of laypeople. In Costa Rica, the example of Dr. Moreno

Cañas, a now-dead physician who has emerged as a mythic medical healer, illustrates a response to this loss of control. Dr. Cañas is petitioned through ritual rather than medical means thereby bringing health care back into the popular healing arena. The combining of medical symbols of technological skill with religious intercession has produced a sacred physician, a popular healing saint, who is prayed to for good health and who has a growing number of devotees. Costa Ricans traditionally prayed to the Virgen de Los Angeles, the country's patron saint, for health and success; her role is now shared with the doctor and his biomedical skills. The recruitment of medical symbols into the ritual and religious system suggests that there is also a pattern of demedicalization generated by the needs of laypeople for sacred explanation and personalized versions of health care.

Medicalization is affecting all aspects of health belief and behavior, and most significantly, is increasing patient reliance on the urban-based, hospital clinics for primary health care and consultation. Casas and Vargas report a rate of medical consultation and drug use similar to developed industrial countries (1980: 264). Cultural medicalization, the incorporation of basic societal functions into the realm of medical control, is an expansion of this process which has influenced the development of a national health care system. Based on the financial success of the Social Security agency in providing health care at low cost, the Costa Rican government mandated that Social Security take over control of all public hospitals and clinics in the country. By nationalizing health care into one system, the provision of medical services is more efficient and financially sound, but nationalization also reduces the number of options in seeking acceptable health care. The rigidity or conflicts of any one system will now affect the health care of the entire nation.

Current reports of the consequences of the reorganization of health care services suggest that "Costa Rica's health performance is impressive" (Harrison 1981: 14) but that the financial burden of the extensive welfare programs since 1976 has created an economic crisis with skyrocketing inflation and a collapse of the government's ability to borrow through its inability to meet foreign debt payments (Schuster 1981: 1). The 1982 physicians' strike against Social Security, because of inadequate wage increases, further illustrates the difficulty of maintaining financial solvency of large social welfare institutions during periods of economic recession (*La Nación* 1981). Casas and Vargas have concluded that the demands of the Costa Rican social democracy are linked to health care, and that the possibility of a viable

National Health Service depends on the nation's political and economic future (Casas and Vargas 1980).

The shift in Costa Rican health culture to a more medicalized form is part of an overall picture of a rapidly modernizing culture. Costa Rica is changing from a rural, agrarian society to a more urbanized, service and factory-based economy. The successes and setbacks of developing a comprehensive and effective health care program are part of this socioeconomic and political transition.

Costa Rica is the second smallest of the Central American republics, covering 50,900 square kilometers with a 1982 total population of 2,276,676 inhabitants (Departamento de Información Comercial 1982, Jaramillo Antillón 1983). The country is comprised of three distinct physical regions: (1) the cool, central highland, (2) the warm Pacific lowlands and westward mountain slopes with marked wet and dry seasons, and (3) the Caribbean lowlands and eastward-facing escarpments, covered by rain forest. The central highlands consist of a northern volcanic range and southern mountain mass, between which lies the Meseta Central (see map of Costa Rica). Two small basins form the upland Meseta; the higher, eastern one of Cartago (5,000 feet elevation), drains toward the Caribbean and the western lower and larger basin of San José (3,000 to 4,000 feet in elevation), drains toward the Pacific. The location of the Meseta Central in the *tierra templada* altitudinal zone benefits from the equable climate and the highly fertile volcanic soil which produces a wide range of crops and supports a dense population (West and Augelli 1966). Over half the population of Costa Rica is concentrated on this highland plateau in communities ranging in density from 300 up to 1,500 inhabitants per square mile (James 1959).

The population of Costa Rica is predominantly (97%) white and Spanish-speaking, with a 2% English-speaking West Indian black segment confined mainly to former banana lands on the Caribbean coast, and 1% indigenous population found in enclaves of the Guatuso, Bribri, Boruca, Térraba, and Cabecar found in the Talamanca region and in other marginal areas of Costa Rica (Chaves Camacho 1969; Hill 1973; West and Augelli 1966; Adams 1956). With the exception of the northwestern province of Guanacaste, Costa Rica remains outside the preconquest cultural influence of Mesoamerica; the indigenous heritage and admixture common in most of Central America, especially Guatemala, El Salvador and western Nicaragua, is absent. The Chibchan, a South American group who had lived in the Meseta Central, resisted colonization and were virtually eliminated with the arrival of the Spanish. Costa Rica's cultural homogeneity, then, centers on the white Spanish-speaking population that dominates the densely settled Meseta Central.

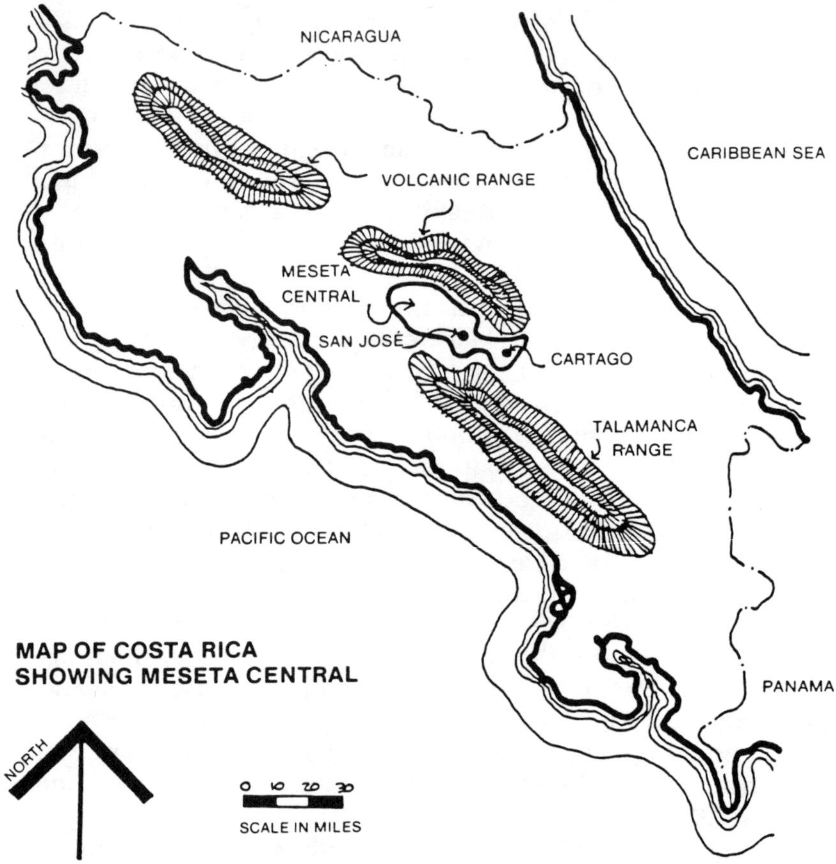

MAP OF COSTA RICA SHOWING MESETA CENTRAL

Costa Rica's agrarian capitalist economy is based on major exports of coffee, bananas, cattle, and sugar (Ministerio de Economía, Industria y Comercio 1970); however, a diminishing proportion of workers participate in the agricultural sector. As a percentage of the active population, 36.7% work as agriculturalists (a drop from almost 50 percent in 1963), 12.0% as service employees, 11.9% as workers in industry and small factories, 8.3% work as professionals and technicians, 5.7% as office employees, 7.4% as businessmen, 4.9% as journeymen and 13.0% in other categories. The surge in world coffee prices during the early 1970s, which stimulated the expansion of social welfare and health care services, increased per capita GNP (as of 1977) to US $ 1240, but did not modify the economy itself (Kane 1979). However the value of their high per capita income is rapidly decreasing as the Costa Rican *colon* is devalued and the rate of inflation approaches 60 percent; increasing unemployment, officially reported at 8.4 percent but calculated at near 12 percent and rising, further threatens an earlier picture of economic stability (Schuster 1981). By 1983 per capita income rose to $1730, but at the same time inflation increased to 120% such that 70% of Costa Ricans could not afford the basic food basket required for adequate nutrition (Castro, personal communication).

There is considerable range in income and education, from a laborer who picks coffee and does odd jobs to the medical doctor or successful San José businessman, yet universal education, a 90% literacy rate, and the vocabulary of cultural belief based on Catholicism and agrarian ideals reduces the social impact of these discrepancies compared to that found in neighboring countries. The increasing separation of the rural agricultural and urban industrial population is more in terms of their differences of world view through unequal access to services and travel opportunities or in terms of the material quality of their lives. At the same time continuity of language and culture does provide a basis for communication across the occupational and class barriers.

Population residence also reflects the decreasing importance of agriculture in Costa Rican life. Of the 60% of the total population that live in rural areas, according to the last census, 84% reside in the same *canton* in which they were born (Ministerio de Economía, Industria y Comercio, Dirección General de Estadística y Censo 1974). The remaining rural sector, therefore, can be described as relatively stable, maintaining local community ties, and established agricultural families. It is predicted, however, that by the year 2000, internal immigration and growth will result in a population that is 75–90% urban (Acuna 1980: 19).

Costa Rica's age pyramid reflects a common Latin American pattern of a large portion (44%) of the population under 15 years of age (Figure I); according to Dwight Heath: "too young to be economically productive and yet they are 'consumers' of costly schooling, health services and so forth" (Heath 1974: 230). In 1959 Costa Rica had a crude live birth rate of 48.3 per 1,000 with a moderate death rate of 9.3 per 1,000 resulting in a rate of increase of 3.9%, one of the highest in the world. The mushrooming population burden was predicted to stress the economy and drastically reduce the quality of life (Newman and Newman 1974: 1). By 1972, however, the birthrate had declined to 31.5 per 1,000, a 35% reduction, and has continued to drop to 28.5 per 1,000 in 1973, although it rose again to 32 per 1,000 in 1978 (Harrison 1981: 15).

This decreasing birth rate is seen at its peak in the narrow 0–4 year category of the age-pyramid for 1973 (Figure I). The explanation for the rapid decline in population growth has been attributed to a number of factors including increased urbanization, changing job structure, increased age at marriage due to land shortage, and more recently, to the widespread availability of birth control and contraceptive acceptance (Low 1977, Thein 1979). According to the World Fertility Survey report, more than three-fourths of all women in unions are currently using contraception (Kane 1979). The 1978 increase was due primarily to delayed marriage and a changing age structure (Harrison 1981: 15).

At the same time that there have been declining birth rates, mortality has also dropped from 9.4 per 1,000 in 1963 to 6.6 per 1,000 in 1972 and finally to 4.3 per 1,000 in 1978 (Bermúdez and Gómez 1974; Harrison 1981: 14). The resulting annual rate of growth of 2.5–2.6 percent for 1978 is slightly above the reported Latin American mean rate of 2.3–2.4 percent (U.S. Bureau of the Census 1980). The varying pressures of population growth and rural, agricultural sector decline influenced family structure and the domestic life cycle as Costa Rican family formation has responded to social change.

Costa Rica is a family based culture. Family and kinship are the major organizing principles in social intercourse; kinship networks when supplemented by friendship and neighborhood ties describe the Costa Rican social world. According to Wolf and Hansen, Latin Americans rely on the more intimate ties of kinship, friendship, and personal acquaintance to provide a buffer against economic scarcity and political uncertainty. They suggest that these kin networks are greatest among the rich and contract within families who possess less wealth and power (1972: 200). The Costa Rican family conforms to the pattern of social relationships which emphasizes family and kin alliances; however, neither the solidarity nor the size of the kinship networks appears to decrease in relation to income. To the contrary, many of the largest kin groups were found among the urban poor and landless rural families. In Costa Rica, as in other parts of Latin America, economic and social power is based on the number of individuals the family can call upon for assistance and support. The poor family is the most economically vulnerable

FIGURE I

Sex-Age Distribution for Costa Rica 1973

Percentages of Total Population

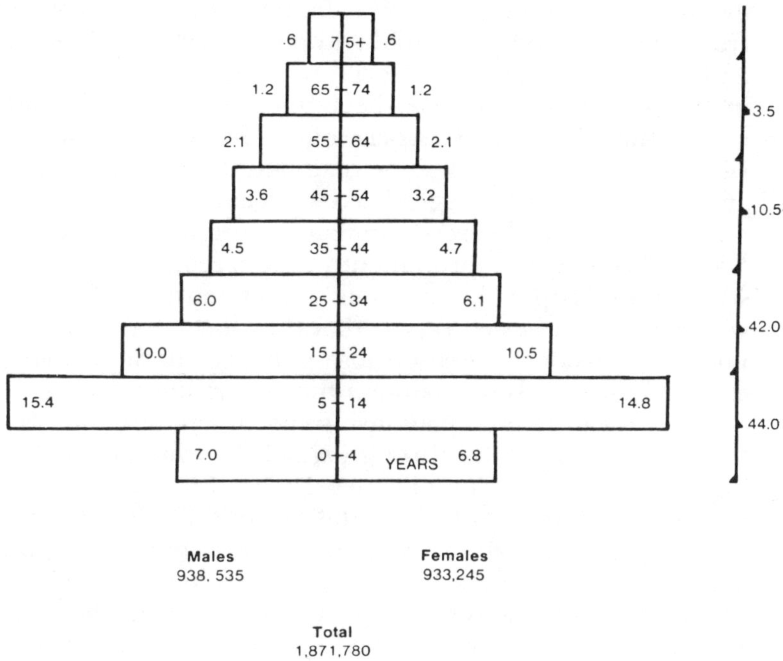

Calculated after: Ministerio de Economía, Industria Y Comercio, Dirección General de Estadistica Y Censos, 1974a. Censo de Población, 1973, Tomo I, San José, Costa Rica.

and therefore has the greatest need to recruit and maintain a cohesive extended family unit. The upper class family network is politically more important and a family member stands to gain power and prestige by affiliation, but economic interdependency is an equally persuasive social force and creates similar social bonding and family organization.

The factors that do appear to influence the degree of solidarity in kin relations are social mobility of the nuclear family and social conflict for deviation from the ideal family model. The households with reduced or minimally functioning kinship networks are those trying to improve their social status or who have come into conflict with parents over some broken social norm: a pregnancy before marriage, a divorce, or abandoning one's child to live with an alcoholic boyfriend.

Urban families are individuated, that is separated and differentiated as distinct autonomous social groups with no encapsulating group or institution that mediates between the family and the total society (Bott 1955). The more individuated a family—in Costa Rica those nuclear families that have broken away from the extended household and particularly the single parent and child—the looser the social network, the less the overlap in network members, and the higher number of friendships rather than kin-linked associations. The women and couples who live in the parental home maintain their tight kin network, and participate in sex-segregated work and family-centered recreation. For the divorced woman or single parent, however, friends become very prominent in their relationships as a substitute for disrupted kin relations. The majority of Costa Ricans who when interviewed report that they have no friends and do not trust outsiders are also those persons who live in large extended households or maintain the closest kin relations.

Costa Rican family relationships are maintained by social interaction, the medium through which bonding, decision-making, and conflict occur (Turner 1970). The pattern of social interaction resembles that of the potter's family described by May Diaz for Tonalá, Mexico: the spheres of males and females are strictly separate, statuses are arranged hierarchically by age, and the locus of power and authority resides in the male and responsibility in the female (1970). These sexually segregated relationships reinforce the separation of the marital and parental aspects of family functioning. The bond between mother and child becomes the primary axis of a family (Peattie 1970). In Costa Rica this primary relationship defines a girl as a woman responsible for the welfare of her child. It is not until a woman has established a recognized sexual relationship through legal, religious, or social means that a separate conjugal household is formed.

If the financial means are not available to acquire a home, the couple may remain in either of the parents' homes, usually that which is most economically capable of providing space and work possibilities. A favorite story of the early years of a marriage is that of mother-in-law and daughter-in-law conflict, especially when the husband's mother is old and alone and the young wife must compete with the intense mother-son relation. One woman complains: "at the time my husband was running around and my mother-in-law antagonized me, mistreated the children. She wanted a girlfriend for my son saying that he was so handsome that he should have lots of children." Another informant reports that they live with her mother-in-law because she "can't live any other place" but that the informant cries all the time because the mother-in-law interferes with their married life. This situation is not considered optimal and usually ends with the separation of the triad. Living with one's mother-in-law is often referred to as a cause of illness.

Family form in Costa Rica varies greatly, producing a wide range of family structure types. Each family type is adaptive in the sense of providing a social context and a set of affiliative relations for its members. The extended family, for example, provides the necessary support when the new mother has inadequate economic and social resources to fulfill her role responsibilities. In situations of severe economic scarcity however, the extended family no longer seems adequate to supply sufficient economic support. The mother-child unit becomes too costly a burden to be sustained by the kin group and other alternatives are sought, as in the following case where the woman and her children live with her employer:

> The informant is a 29 year old woman, a domestic with two children by two different fathers. The fathers will not help with the support of the children. She lived two years with her first boyfriend but when she got pregnant he left her. Her parents live in the next community. She is happy with the woman she works for (as a live-in domestic) but she is not paid a wage, only given room and board. She needs money for the little boy and baby girl. When asked why she doesn't live with her mother she says that her family cannot support her; that they are very poor. (Fieldnotes 1973)

Other interviews indicate that children are sometimes permanently left with their maternal grandparents while the mother pursues new relationships which do stabilize and eventually form nuclear families. In most cases it was the first born who was adopted, usually when the mother was quite young and her employment opportunities restricted by the presence of the child.

A family cycle is thus described in which a woman may have a child while living with her parents, and later marry and move out to form a nuclear household. Siblings or other family members may then move in with the new family in periods of economic and social stress. The offspring upon maturity may marry or have children before forming a separate household to repeat the cycle. The variation of family composition therefore is an artifact of this developmental cycle.

Recent modification of the family law of Costa Rica indicates that family structure has changed and women's legal position has improved. In the original code, the husband supplied the income, controlled all property, and initiated divorce. Because of the lower fertility of women and their subsequent increased participation in industry and higher education, these laws are no longer adequate. The new family code extends women's legal property and earning rights and expands the basis for divorce to include adultery of either partner and legally declared conjugal absence as reasonable cause; in other words, a woman may divorce a man for his *casa chica* (the ubiquitous Latin American mistress), or for his prolonged absence through neglect or migrant working conditions. The new code also undermines the inviolate parental control of children, by declaring that a doctor can perform surgery necessary to save a child's life without parental permission (*Asamblea Legislativa* 1974). These changes will influence cultural patterns of sex role behavior and responsibility. Even at the level of the family, Costa Rican culture is undergoing change.

San José: Urbanization and Social Change

The process of change also can be seen in the growth, urbanization, and socioeconomic development of Costa Rica's capital city, San José, located in the center of the Meseta Central (see map). San José is home for 53% of the country's total urban population (Ministerio de Economía, Industria y Comercio, Dirección General de Estadística y Censos 1974). Its metropolitan population of over 460,000 represented one fourth of the nation's total population in the last available census count (1973). By 1983, the total urban population had increased to 1,001,738 or 44% of the entire country (Jaramillo Antillón 1983). San José's rapid urbanization is disrupting the fabric of traditional Costa Rican life and changing the relationship of individuals to social institutions.

Historically, San José was first mentioned in 1708 as a nuclear population which did not fulfill its obligation to the Catholic Church (de Mora 1973). In 1736 a mandate by the Church brought the dispersed population together and authorized a chapel to be built, forming the parish of Villa Nueva de la Boca del Monte, consisting of 399 families or 2,330 persons without counting indigenous settlement (Calvo 1887). These families were descendants of the early Spanish settlers who migrated to the New World following the discovery of Costa Rica in 1508 by Columbus at Cariay (present-day Puerto Limon on the Atlantic Coast). Although granted *encomienda* rights (rights to labor and land granted by the Spanish crown to individuals in the

New World) and duties, the small indigenous population did not provide an adequate labor force for large land holdings and most colonists were occupied with subsistence farming (MacLeod 1973; Monge Alfaro 1974). Political posts, however, continued to be awarded to "a small group of families by virtue of their descent" (Stone 1974: 406) which enabled this group to monopolize cacao cultivation and later coffee production.

Population growth was stimulated first by the 1789–90 tobacco harvest and the building of a tobacco factory, and later by the introduction of coffee at the turn of the century (Seligson 1974). The importation from Cuba and distribution of 300 trees in San Vicente by Presbitero Felix Velarde in 1815 produced an excellent harvest and began the characteristic landscape of

> land covered with the rich coffee plantation of San José... laid out into squares of two hundred feet and enclosed by living fences of trees bearing flowers. (Stephens 1949: 284)

By 1844 San José had grown to over 20,000 persons under the impetus of both Costa Rica's separation from Spain in 1821 and its designation as the capital of the new republic in 1828 (Bustamante Guerrero de Rivera 1961; de Mora 1973). An 1853 traveler describes the city as:

> ...the only city that has grown up or even improved since the independence of Central America. Under the Spanish dominion Cartago was the royal capital; but, on the breaking out of the revolution, the fervor of patriotism was so hot that it resolved to abolish this memorial to colonial servitude and to establish the capital at San José. Their local advantages are perhaps equal. Cartago is nearer the Atlantic, San José the Pacific, but they are only six leagues apart. The buildings in San José are all republican; not one is of any grandeur or architectural beauty, and the churches are inferior to many erected by the Spaniards in the smallest villages. Nevertheless, it exhibited a development of resources and an appearance of business unusual in this lethargic country. (Stephens 1949: 289).

Stephens attributes this prosperity and growth to Costa Rica's lack of indigenous labor and mineral wealth which encouraged the development of a large class of industrious yeomen farmers. It was not until the introduction of agrarian capitalism and the advent of coffee production that major economic differences would change social relationships and divide Costa Rica into the landed and landless (Seligson 1980).

San José continues to grow at an accelerated rate (calculated to be a mean annual increase of 5.3% from 1970 to 1973) double that for the country as a whole (2.7% for the same period). This urban growth is essentially maintained by the absorption of the surrounding ring of autonomous communities by the expanding city. The urban settlement pattern gradually merges into the countryside creating a transitional sector inhabited by an agriculturally based subculture which acts as a buffer delaying urban acculturation, although not halting the exploitation of city services (Willems 1968; Solis Zeledon et al. 1969). San José is the center of economic, political, and social networks and of decision-making, representing all levels of organization and power (Leeds 1968). The capital acts as a centralizing force for the majority of Costa Ricans who live in localities with populations less than 1,000 inhabitants. All major social institutions, including hospitals and clinics, are located in San José. It is here under the pressure of rapid urbanization and increasing bifurcation of the class structure that the impact of social change on institutions can be examined through the major medical institutions that developed in response to the changing socioeconomic and political structures.

The Development of Medical Institutions

The Public Health and Social Security agencies provide the majority of hospital care available in Costa Rica. The development of these medical institutions began with the advent of a coffee-based economy. The first charity institution was founded in Cartago in 1781 and completed in 1815 by Obispo Tristán to house the sick, wounded, demented, orphans, and lepers of Costa Rican society. In 1826, a Constitutional Assembly decree was passed, providing for the founding of a general hospital in San José. In 1845, Dr. José María Castro began La Junta de Caridad, a government agency for the administration of charity, and Hospital San Juan de Dios was constructed beginning in 1852. Its doors were opened by the Sisters of Charity, with the support of the executive government in 1863 (Schapiro 1962: 492–4). In 1923 a secretariat was established placing the hospital under the auspices of the Ministry of Public Health (Monge Alfaro 1974).

Tension had developed in Costa Rica as a result of labor conflicts in the 1920s and 1930s (Seligson 1980). During the 1930s the Communists, under the competent and respected leadership of Manuel Mora Valverde, gained considerable strength and established themselves as the national ideological party (Bell 1971). When Dr. Calderon Guardia (president of Costa Rica 1940–44) lost the support of many elite and white-collar groups because of confused public administration and pro-labor policies, his party had to rely more heavily on Mora's Communist influenced and operated labor union, Vanguardia Popular and its supporters (Denton 1971). The Social Security was created in 1941 both in response to Calderon Guardia's interest in elite social reform, and in exchange for the political support of Mora in the Legislative Assembly (Caja Costarricense de Seguro 1972; Rosenberg 1981). In 1942 the medical institution began to provide illness and maternity insurance in San José, and in 1943 the Labor Code was completed, consolidating a number of health and social welfare guarantees (Bell 1971). Disability, old age, and death insurance was extended to specific occupational groups in 1947. Subsequent Social Security laws and modifications both raised the deductions and progressively extended services to an increasing proportion of workers and, in 1948, to their families (Caja Costarricense de Seguro Social 1972).

The final stage in the development of Costa Rican medical institutions was the passage of the 1973 law which transferred the economic and administrative control of the Public Health hospitals and clinics to Social Security. This transfer of power is to take place over a ten year period at which time it is expected that Social Security will be the national health care system. In actuality the government does not have the majority of votes on the governing board, but maintains a voice in the institution's direction. The designation, "semi-autonomous," reflects Social Security's legal and financial status with relation to the public (government) and private (business) sectors.

The development of medical institutions could not have been possible without the complementary development of a legitimized group of medical practitioners. Throughout the colonial period, medical practitioners functioned without licenses reportedly causing complaints of high prices and questionable curing success (Von Bulow 1974: 138). Upon the arrival of the first licensed physician in 1781, a division developed between licensed and unlicensed practitioners. The first legal case against a curer practicing without a license was instigated soon after (Schapiro 1962). The tension between licensed and unlicensed practitioners in Costa Rica has continued, and is reflected in the law which declares homeopaths and other paramedical practitioners illegal. With the legal exclusion of paramedical practitioners, the biomedical physicians have been able to maintain professional control of the medical field.

The role of the doctor in Costa Rica is highly prestigious, and associated with high social status and political leverage. Doctors historically were sons of the upper class, educated abroad, who upon their return practiced medicine and participated in politics. Currently many Costa Rican physicians are trained at the Universidad de Costa Rica, and begin their practice locally, still maintaining socially powerful networks and political relationships. A number of Costa Rican presidents have been physicians with reputations as charitable individuals who generate a large following. The role and social position of the physician is one avenue to political power, combining personal prestige with an upper class family name and social dedication to create a charismatic personage. Drs. Calderon Guardia, José María Castro, José María Montealegre, Carlos Duran, and Vicente Herrera are examples of successful doctors who became presidents of the republic.

In the medical anthropological literature there is also evidence of the importance of the physician in both Latin American and North American culture. Myerhoff (1965), using the portrayal of doctors on North American television, suggests that the physician is a cultural hero embodying the morality and personality most valued by American society. Bertrand and Micklin (1979), in a recent article that statistically reviews the influence of and preference for physicians over other health practitioners, point out that there is little doubt of the overwhelming prestige of the physician in Latin America and little evidence that any other category of practitioner will supplant his dominant position. Denton (1971) in *Costa Rican Politics* has pointed out that doctors play a major role in the political arena and will continue to do so.

The development of medical institutions and a large physician population combined with a community health care system has contributed to the fact that Costa Rica enjoys impressively high levels of health and medical care. According to Paul Harrison of *World Health*, Costa Rica now reports among the lowest mortality rate in the world (4.3 per 1000), an infant mortality rate of 22 per 1000 which is below Eastern European levels, and a life expectancy of 72.3, which is on a level with Great Britain. Further, measles, diphtheria, and polio have been significantly reduced by vaccination programs and malaria has been eliminated since 1968 due to public health programs. Malnutrition is rare; only 9 percent of children had second degree and .3 percent third degree in 1973, compared to the Central American average of 33 percent for second and third degree malnutrition. (1981: 14)

The geographic distribution of physicians within Costa Rica, however, is not equal. For example, between 1960 and 1973 the ratio of physicians per inhabitant doubled. On the other hand, 71.7% of these physicians practice in the metropolitan areas of San José, thus neglecting many rural areas (Bermúdez and Gómez 1974; Gutierrez Saenz 1971). By 1978, 1515 physicians were practicing (7.2 per 1000 population) but with 1 per 200 persons in the capital and 1 per 10,000 on the periphery (Casas and Vargas 1980).

As with many countries experiencing modernization and improved health care, the leading causes of mortality in Costa Rica have changed. As recently as 1969, gastroenteritis and colitis were the principle causes of death in Costa Rica; however, as clean water has reached three-quarters of the population, diarrhea has dropped from their list of top complaints. By 1972, diseases of the circulatory system, and cancers, had assumed preeminence in the Costa Rican mortality pattern (Ministerio de Economía, Industria y Censos, Dirección de Estadística y Censos 1972). Analysis of this pattern by province, however, shows that the lowland coastal areas—the banana and cattle lands—retain the former mortality pattern which emphasizes infectious diseases while the modern pattern characterizes the Meseta Central. With the current nationalization of the health system providing more consistent rural health care, the trend of changing disease pattern of the highlands is spreading to all parts of the country. The *World Health* report identifies the Costa Rican program of preventive health care by rural health workers combined with maternal and child health centers, nutritional programs, and radio health education as an effective model for primary health care (Harrison 1981).

Cultural Medicalization: the Case of Dr. Moreno Cañas

There are few examples other than the case of Dr. Moreno Cañas that so clearly illustrate the dramatic symbolic shift from religious to medical vocabularies of healing in a Latin American population, thereby underscoring the cultural conflicts and ideals surrounding health care in a modernizing world.

Dr. Ricardo Moreno Cañas was born in San José, Costa Rica, the 8th of May, 1890. He attended medical school at the University of Geneva graduating as a medical surgeon in 1915. Moreno Cañas returned to Costa Rica in 1920 as a medical intern at San Juan de Dios, the major public hospital facility in the country. In 1923 he was named surgical assistant, and in 1927 became chief of the Department of Orthopedics, a department which he had created, bringing scientific practices previously unknown to this important branch of surgical services. At first his efforts met with hostility from his peers, but with continued work and clinical demonstration of the success of his direction, Orthopedics became an acclaimed department.

In 1936 Dr. Moreno Cañas was named the Chief of Surgery for the entire hospital. He had developed an enormous reputation and large patient following; his dedication and hard work won him recognition as a major figure and the most reknowned surgeon of his generation. A recent editorial quotes Dr. Peña Chavarría as saying that Dr. Moreno Cañas' name stood out to the point of being considered a candidate for the Presidency of the Republic. His performance of open heart surgery in 1934 was widely publicized, brought him international acclaim, and is still remembered with great admiration (El Seguro 1980: 6).

On the night of August 23, 1938, Drs. Ricardo Moreno Cañas and Carlos Manuel Echandi were assassinated in their homes by an ex-patient. When apprehended by the authorities, the assassin justified his act by stating that his arm had been left deformed by an unsuccessful operation on a fractured humerus performed in the charity clinic of San Juan de Dios by the two doctors over seven years before. The news announcement decried the crime as a "symptom of the cancer of society which would ultimately destroy the moral structure of the country" (El Seguro 1980: 6).

Dr. Moreno Cañas is still viewed by Costa Ricans as a healer. The published literature does not indicate how soon after his demise individuals began to petition him for medication and healing, but by 1973 during interviews with patients concerning their health care practices, interviewees were either using his name, or viewing him in some healing capacity. The general explanation by a Costa Rican petitioner is that Dr. Moreno Cañas can intervene directly as he was such a fine doctor and would know which medication or technique would truly work. The interview data suggest that individuals of various social and economic backgrounds, ages, and of both sexes, believe in the Doctor's ability to effect cures.

Interviewees report to have experienced a cure by Dr. Moreno Cañas through a number of different avenues:

1. Through direct personal experience with him while he was alive.
2. Through petitions to him by prayer or the recitation of a formula which can be purchased in religious devotion shops in the central market.

3. Through the use of a glass of water and a cut lemon cross which are laid out with a prayer that invites the doctor to visit the house and give the patient the proper healing medicine to be drunk out of the glass in the morning.
4. Through a partial apparition of the doctor's hand or coat in response to a petitioner's request.
5. Through a total apparition in which the doctor is said to visit the patient carrying a black bag, often accompanied by his nurse, in order to examine and/or operate on the petitioner to cure the illness or correct the physical disorder.
6. Through spiritual contact with the doctor by means of a medium through whom the doctor can speak with the patient and give instructions for treatment.

Examples of each kind of intervention or some combination of the above are presented in Chapter II.

The important anthropological and sociological issue in the case of Dr. Moreno Cañas is why this one figure of the historical past has become such a focus for Costa Ricans. Certainly, there are other persons and saints to whom Costa Ricans could pray and petition health and good fortune. For example, Costa Ricans have a long history of patronage to the Virgen de Los Angeles who has been the patron saint of that country since 1824.

An explanation for the cultural choice of Dr. Moreno Cañas as a popular image is his symbolic linkage to modern technology and foreign culture. His education in Switzerland conforms with the Costa Rican belief that a better life and material wealth come from outside the country. As in many parts of Latin America, Costa Ricans are increasing their consumption of manufactured goods. The resulting economic and cultural dependence on European and North American countries has considerable influence on the ideas and choices made by Costa Ricans in their daily lives. Dr. Moreno Cañas' professional choice of orthopedics carried with it the dramatic quality of surgical intervention accompanied by high technology machinery and complicated biomedical procedures.

Another way to approach the issue of why Dr. Moreno Cañas has gained such popularity is to examine the national transition from religious to biomedical institutions of medical care. Costa Rica is experiencing secularization which has steadily increased the power of the state in the management of national affairs. This secularization began in the 1850s with the expulsion of the Jesuits and is reflected in the sponsorship of the hospital system which was once in the hands of the clergy but then passed to the young, upper-class legislators in the 1920 legislative assembly. By 1940, a government sponsored health and social security system was begun, which was nationalized with mandatory enrollment in 1974.

The secularization of health care has been accompanied by a corresponding process of desacralization in which religious concepts and treatment of disease are replaced by secular ones. For instance, interviews with Costa Rican psychiatric administrators indicate that there is a growing reliance on psychiatrists over religious curers in the treatment of mental problems. From 1963 to 1973, the number of psychiatrists increased from six to forty (Interview 1973). That is not to say that curers are not used, but an increasing number of patients now go to Hospital Chapui, the national mental health hospital, for medication and psychological consultation. The head of psychiatric services in an urban clinic asserts that ten years ago only 30% of all patients were self-referred for psychiatric services; now 90% of all patients come on their own. This change in attitude and increased utilization of psychiatric services suggests that mental illness, which was traditionally defined and treated within the religious domain, is now referred to the professional medical sector. Mental illness more frequently is perceived as a disease of the head or nerves rather than a punishment for religious transgressions.

The lay response to the secularization/desacralization process has been to incorporate symbolic elements from the secular medical world. Dr. Moreno Cañas, a physician, has been transformed into a sacred symbol, a secular saint, and treated by cult participants with ritual behaviors similar to those accorded to the Virgen de Los Angeles. There are parallels in the symbolic expression of popular healing attributed to both of them. They are indigenous figures who were seen in Costa Rica by local people thus representing nationalism and patriotic pride. Both figures cure, bring good luck, and may intercede directly with God who has the ultimate control. A petition to either may be a plea that the individual will speak to God and obtain the necessary request or the request may be for direct intervention. The difference is in the symbolic system by which the healing message is expressed. The Virgen de Los Angeles is an aspect of the many manifestations of the Virgin Mary. Her national importance is enhanced by her symbolic linkage to the Latin American Catholic Church. Dr. Moreno Cañas, on the other hand represents the secular, biomedical, and political world of Costa Rica. His recruitment into a cult which employs religious rituals for healing illustrates the sacralization of medical symbols, a part of the lay response to the medicalization of health care.

The symbolic importance of the medicalization process is corroborated by the response of patients to the change in Costa Rican health care from a charity/public health system to a nationalized social security system. The resulting bureaucratization and depersonalization of health care has increased the symbolic relevance of a figure like Dr. Moreno Cañas, who reflects an earlier period of health care characterized by a paternalistic relationship between the doctor and the patient. Dr. Moreno Cañas represents both an idealized version of traditional healing style and a role model of a physician that Costa Ricans can understand and respect. Social Security doctors who attempt to treat their patients as social equals create a confusion in interactional style which reduces patient satisfaction with treatment and medical consultation. This idealized physician model is a reassuring healing alternative as the relationship between real doctors and patients deteriorates because of the growing size of medical institutions and increasing impersonality of the health care delivery system.

CHAPTER II

THE URBAN PATIENT

The Urban Health Care System

The description of the urban health care system, as it exists in San José, requires a typology of medical beliefs and practices which defines coexisting sectors of a socially complex and pluralistic medical situation. Kleinman proposes that these sectors are "professional", "popular" and "folk" medicine; "three social arenas within which sickness is experienced and reacted to" (1978: 86). Press, in his critique of medical system typologies, comments that "the differences between these three sectors are anything but clear" (1980: 48) and suggests that we should standardize our use of these categories by referring to the systems or practices of medicine in terms of their dominance within a particular culture or society. In Costa Rica, then, professional medicine, the official or accepted medical paradigm, is defined as Western biomedicine; popular medicine includes both officially sanctioned medical practices performed outside the professional medical setting, and family-based beliefs and practices which originate in the home with traditional or indigenous origins; while folk medicine refers to systems or practices which differ from those of the dominant system.

For the purposes of this discussion the typology is viewed from the perspective of the patient. For the urban patient, professional medicine is practiced in hospitals and clinics. Popular medicine begins at home and extends to health-seeking behaviors which derive from family and community efforts at self-care and home treatment. Folk medicine is practiced by a variety of specialists located in the community who represent a range of indigenous and foreign healing expertise.

The presentations of the three medical sectors are based on

overlapping sources of descriptive data. The professional medicine sector is described through the observed clinic consultations from the perspective of the patient. The popular sector description is based on interviews and observations of pharmacy clients in locations scattered throughout the city. The discussion of Dr. Moreno Cañas and the Virgen de Los Angeles is based on home interviews, ethnographic accounts, and observation in the Basilica de Nuestra Señora de Los Angeles located in Cartago, Costa Rica. Finally, the folk sector data are from a study by Dr. María Eugenia Bozzoli de Wille supplemented by home interviews, market excursions and references to folk medical practices recorded during medical consultations. By employing materials from both primary and secondary sources a more complete description of the health care system of San José has been possible.

Professional Medicine: Public Health and Social Security Outpatient Clinics

Professional medicine in San José is a complex system of overlapping public, quasi-public, and private hospitals and clinics. Over 1,200 physicians work in these institutions, providing patient care in large hospital outpatient clinics until late afternoon and then seeing private patients in small offices throughout the early evening. Often the patients are the same having been referred by the physician from the larger clinics for a more intensive work-up in private consultation.

San José medical institutions include the Public Health hospitals and clinics, the Social Security hospitals and clinics, the National Insurance Institute hospital, and private hospitals serving the American missionary and wealthy Catholic populations. Private offices provide a number of specialty clinics as well as a few practitioners of chiropractic and osteopathic medicine. These offices and hospitals are spread throughout the urban neighborhoods serving a diverse population of patients seeking professional medical care. Professional medicine is dominated by the Western biomedical physicians trained in Costa Rica, Mexico, the United States, and Europe who practice in these medical institutions.

It is difficult to represent the entire professional medical sector in any detail and at the same time fully cover the breadth of practitioners and office settings. Therefore, the professional sector is presented as characterized by the research sample observed in the Public Health and Social Security outpatient clinics. These clinics are utilized by a majority of San José residents and provide the broadest possible descriptions of a cross-section of urban patients. Most patients at least start the medical institutional phase of their health seeking in these clinics, even if they are later advised to return to the physician's private practice for personal advice and further treatment.

The clinic sample employed to describe the professional sector consists of 457 patients observed in matched clinics in the two major medical institutions (see Figure II). Each sample represents 1 to 7% of the monthly consultations recorded at each clinic in 1973. In the Ministry of Public Health hospital, San Juan de Dios, 101 observations were collected in the *consulta extemporanea*—the outpatient service where patients receive immediate treatment without appointments for minor illnesses, referrals to specialty clinics, or are hospitalized—and 50 observations in the *consulta externa*—the general medicine outpatient service which requires appointments and where patients are followed by their own doctors. Fifty-one *consulta extemporanea* and 103 *consulta externa* outpatients were also observed in the Social Security hospital, Calderon Guardia, and 50 collected from the psychosomatic outpatient clinic in Hospital Mexico of the Social Security system; the psychosomatic and psychiatric clinics overlap in function and compete for patients, therefore both clinics were investigated. Because of the large number of patient observations, statistical comparisons were used whenever possible to distinguish patient characteristics.

The research sample was 67.7% female and 32.3% male. The high percentage of female clinic attendance may be explained by a number of factors of sample selection and cultural patterning: 1) most men work during the day when clinics were observed; 2) patients are often accompanied by their mothers who also seek care, thereby increasing the total number of female patients observed; and 3) there is a cultural expectation in Costa Rica that men should endure illness and injury while women freely express their physical difficulties which could influence clinic attendance. Clinic observation and patient interviews suggest that women also use the clinic experience as a social occasion where they can visit with friends, gossip and watch the on-going hospital drama.

Patient ages were coded into five groups: those under 15 years of age represented 17% of observed clinical consultations; 15 to 30 years—31.7%; 31 to 45 years—25.7%; 46 to 60 years—16.6%; and over 60 years—9.0%. The mean patient age was 33.5 years, and over half of the patients were young adults (aged 15–45). Teller (1972) similarly reports that young adults (aged 15 to 44) had the highest access rates, utilizing both public and private clinics, in San Pedro Sula, Honduras. Infants and young

FIGURE II

Distribution of Patient Samples By Institution, Hospitals, & Services

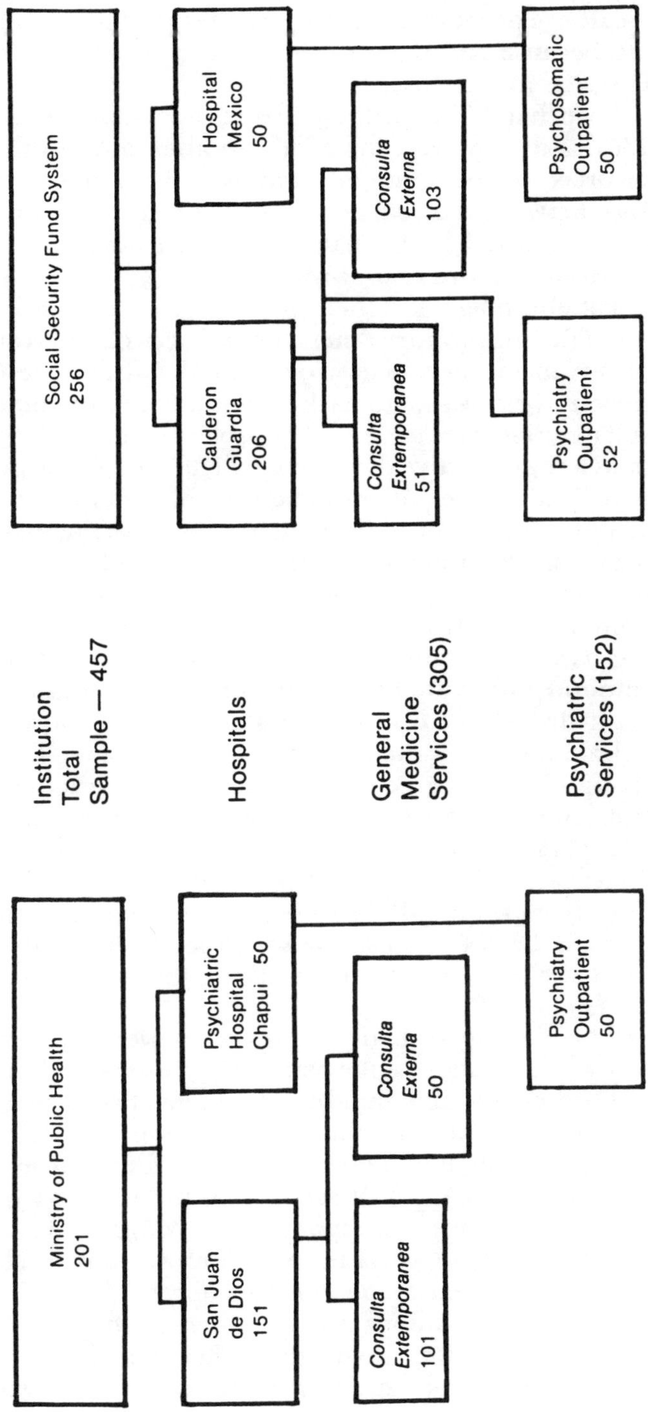

children, who in developing countries have a relatively high incidence of morbidity, are underrepresented in the clinic sample because the majority of these cases go to the Children's Hospital in San José.

Over half, 56%, of the patients reporting marital status (n = 134) said they were married, another 30% were single, 10% divorced or separated, 4% widowed, with no significant difference between medical institutions. The average number of children reported by 98 patients was 4.3 with a range from no children to more than 9 recorded.

Patients diagnosed their problems to the physician most often as: minor respiratory illness (*grippe*), a problem from their work or advancing age, a gastrointestinal disturbance (*bichos*, parasites; *mal estomago*, stomach ache), a result of some kind of accident or blow (*golpe*), a social problem (such as alcohol or abuse), or as a reproductive dysfunction (Table I). These problems were perceived by the patient to be precipitated by a spouse's illness, abandonment, abuse or drinking behavior; by paternal or maternal abuse or abandonment; maternal illness; reduced affect or disciplinary action; abuse from one's children or siblings; and economic family problems. These patient complaints represent the basic emic categories of Costa Rica illness and in fact correspond rather well to the major kinds of disease which exist according to medical and epidemiological sources. The etiological reasons for the development of these medical complaints, though, do not agree with Western biomedical theory and practice. Their explanations for illness are predominantly social and interpersonal conflicts, while physician's explanations tend to focus on underlying biophysical processes. The conflicts that arise from these differences of perspective are somewhat ameliorated by the medicalization process which affects patients' health behavior and the cultural continuity of Costa Rican health culture.

The majority of patients previously were treated in the same medical institution; some patients had used the alternate medical institution as well; a number of patients had seen a private doctor, been to the pharmacy, tried a home remedy, visited the emergency room of a hospital, or seen a folk curer for the same complaint (Table II). It seems that the diversity of complaints and explanations corresponds to a complex health care utilization pattern which is presented more fully in a later section based on detailed home interview material.

Patient expectations are described in the literature as those qualities desired in the doctor rather than in terms of the outcome of the consultation or an evaluation of dissatisfaction. A

Table I
Patients' Diagnosis of Complaints

Patient Diagnosis	*Absolute Frequency*	*Relative Frequency (Percent)*	*Adjusted Frequency (Percent)*
Minor Respiratory	23	5.0	10.1
Work or Age Related	22	4.8	9.6
Gastrointestinal	20	4.4	8.8
Social Problem	17	3.7	7.5
Accident	17	3.7	7.5
Reproductive System Related	14	3.1	6.1
Well or Cured	14	3.1	6.1
Endocrine	11	2.4	4.8
Nervios	10	2.2	4.4
Folk Concept	10	2.2	4.4
Dermatological	10	2.2	4.4
Major Respiratory	9	2.0	3.9
Urogenital	7	1.5	3.1
Hereditary Genital	7	1.5	3.1
Other Psychological	7	1.5	3.1
Circulatory	5	1.1	2.2
Neural	5	1.1	2.2
Nutrition Related	4	0.9	1.8
Orthopedic, Osteological	4	0.9	1.8
Neurosis	3	0.7	1.3
Hot-Cold Concept	3	0.7	1.3
Other Systematic	3	0.7	1.3
Sensory Organ	2	0.4	0.9
No Data	230	50.3	Missing
Total	457	100.0	100.0

study of three outpatient clinics in Colombia reveals that patients expressed "dissatisfaction with the physician's lack of empathy" (Ordonez Plaja et. al. 1968: 184). Patients liked a physician who gave them "proper" treatment, who was respectful and courteous. In the United States patients expect doctors to be friendly and concerned, yet only 5% of the doctor-patient interactions fulfill this expectation (Korsch and Negrete 1972: 72). Friedson, in a study of United States medical group care, found that patients wanted: (1) technical adequacy demonstrated by indicators of care and thoroughness such as concrete examinations and laboratory tests, and a diagnosis that fits the patient's own suspicions and confirmation of symptoms and pain; (2) personal interest such as conversation in the consulting room and absence of "mechanical" or "abrupt" behavior; and (3) accessibility in the form of home visits (1963: 60–61).

Table II
Patients' Treatment History for Current Complaint

Treatment	*Absolute Frequency*	*Relative Frequency (Percent)*	*Adjusted Frequency (Percent)*
Same Medical Institution[1]	145	31.7	56.2
Other Medical Institution[2]	32	7.0	12.4
Private Doctor	24	5.3	9.3
Pharmacy	16	3.5	6.2
Home Remedy	10	2.2	3.9
Emergency Room	10	2.2	3.9
Missed Appointment	10	2.2	3.9
Curer[3]	7	1.5	2.7
Nothing	4	0.9	1.6
No Data	199	43.5	Missing
Total	457	100.0	100.0

[1] Refers to a patient report that he/she previously had seen a physician in the same medical institution as the current consultation.

[2] Refers to a patient report that he/she previously had seen a physician in the other medical institution, rather than in the one in which they were currently being treated, i.e. if the patient is being observed in the Public Heath Clinic, the "other medical institution" would be the Social Security clinic and vice versa.

[3] Curer refers here to a range of folk medical practitioners that are called *curanderos* and are discussed in the section on folk medicine.

The Costa Rican patient's expectations, however, do not emphasize concern with physician personality, but focus on treatment and consultation outcome. Clinic patients expected the doctor to give them medicine or tranquilizers, some kind of physical or laboratory examination, or explanation of their illness. They specifically requested medicine, exams, explanation, and referral in the consultation (Table III). The Costa Rican patients generally reported that they were satisfied with the treatment received. According to the national hospital statistics, outpatients at San Juan de Dios and Calderon Guardia do receive an average of two prescriptions each, one-fifth of all patients have x-rays taken, and one-half have clinical laboratory examinations. These prescriptions and exams fulfill patient requests and may account for the informants' elicited satisfaction. Further, studies of consumer assessments from patient interviews usually report about 80% satisfaction on the part of interviewees (Lebow 1974). This conclusion suggests that reports of dissatisfaction are better indicators of the patient's medical experience.

A more detailed examination of the professional medicine patient data reflects variation in style and content of health behavior within the consultation. For instance, male and female patients do not necessarily behave similarly during a medical consultation. In the following two cases, young middle income Costa Ricans both are searching for an explanation of their illness in the general medicine clinic of Calderon Guardia:

> A young woman, attractive with stylish clothes and make-up. She is a school teacher. She begins by saying: "I am ashamed, doctor, I won't take the large pills anymore." She takes the penicillin which is very strong, but when she does, it makes her cough and choke. Her throat is very dry. She asks, "Doctor, what shall I do?" She doesn't and can't take those big pills. They give her a pain in the head. And the cold bothers her because she wears a very light nightgown; she is always cold and this bothers her. What can she do about the phlegm? Other problems are the pain in her head, tiredness and all the time she wants to sleep. Doctor examines the patient; listens to her breathing. She talks as the doctor listens to her chest and asks the doctor to check her heartbeat. She sleeps all day and wonders what is wrong; how did it all start? Doctor replies that she has an inflamation of the throat which is very common in teachers who use the voice a lot. Her lungs are good although she does have spasms of the lungs. She asks how to spell the medical term for spasms of the lungs and writes it down saying that she is trying to learn. The doctor orders medications and suggests further tests. She says goodbye to the doctor and to me.

> Young man in a company uniform. Shakes hands with the doctor and walks over and shakes hands with me. He says that he has been tired for four months and that his stomach hurts. He wasn't sleeping so he self-treated with Valium. Doctor asks what food hurts. He can't answer; doctor lists coffee, cigarettes, hot things. Young man nods and says he has an acid stomach. He also took patent medicine but it hurt his stomach. Doctor tells him he will give him a pill to take before bed and to double the dosage if it doesn't work. The patient goes on asking if he shouldn't see a psychiatrist. Doctor says no, he wants to try the medicine first, and then they will see. Patient then continues that he also has a pain inside of his knee, a little pain (*dolorcito*) in both knees. He had an accident in December and was hit on the head and nose... he thinks that the pain is from there... doesn't he? Doctor examines him again and says that he will refer him to a specialty clinic (internal medicine).

Table III
Patients' Expectations and Requests[1]

Expectations	*N*	*% of all Expectations*
Medicine	62	36.3
Physical or Laboratory Examination	39	22.8
Explanation of Illness	19	11.1
Tranquilizers	18	10.5
Referral	8	4.7
Injection	8	4.7
Incapacidad (Incapacity Petition)	6	3.5
Hospitalization	2	1.2
Other—Don't Know	9	5.3
Total	171	100.0
Requests		
Medicine	48	29.3
Examinations	38	23.2
Explanations	24	14.6
Referral	23	14.0
Hospitalization	10	6.1
Incapacidad	9	5.5
Other	12	7.3
Total	164	100.0

[1] Data obtained from 117 patients by before-and-after consultation interviews conducted consecutively by a research assistant in the waiting room while the author was observing consultations inside the physician's office. Patients frequently expressed more than one expectation or request.

The young woman is talkative and coquettish while the young man is more reserved. This difference in male and female patient style was observed in all clinic settings.

Another male-female difference is illustrated by two ulcer patients at San Juan de Dios:

> A 35 year old woman, a recent migrant from the countryside. Doctor asks before she sits down: "What do you have?" She says that she has an acid stomach and she doesn't know if it is an ulcer. She has pain in her side, both high and low and also has pain in her back. The pain is worse at night. She has a problem with eating. She vomits even when she eats rice with only salt and boiled chayote, things without grease and that are not hot (*picante*). Patient seems to feel pain when the doctor examines her. She grimaces as the doctor pushes on her stomach. She is given another appointment.

> A man of 22 from San José. Says that he has a pain in the mouth of his stomach and is very tired, why doctor? A friend gave him some white liquid to take which did not help. Doctor examines him and patient feels a lot of pain when the doctor examines him. (Doctor says to me that the man has an ulcer.) Patient also complains of a cough. Doctor writes down "duodenal ulcer" and gives the patient a diet, medicines and orders exams including an x-ray of the stomach. Tells him to come back.

The woman is more direct with the doctor; she provides her own diagnosis asking if she has an ulcer, while the man is unaware of what kind of illness he has. She offers specific information concerning her illness and relates her symptoms in greater detail and number. Women present an average of 3.25 symptoms per patient compared to men's 2.75 symptoms per patient, suggesting that women report more symptoms or use a larger number of symptoms to describe their presenting complaint.

Age differences in patient behavior reflect culturally prescribed personality and interaction appropriate to the various stages of the Costa Rican life cycle. Young adult patients, those 15 to 30 years of age, are often reticent with the doctor, unable to request services or demand treatment. Older patients are increasingly aggressive, attempt to control the doctor's care, and suggest possible diagnoses and remedies. Younger patients may try a home remedy before consulting a physician, but older patients are more experienced in medical institution utilization and may have previously consulted a private doctor, pharmacist, and/or curer. Disease patterns vary: younger patients with minor respiratory, gastrointestinal, and dermatological problems, and the older patients with greater chronicity from major respiratory and circulatory disease.

Doctors' explanatory models when elicited in interviews or offered during consultations reveal culturally defined patterns. The younger patients' disturbances are most often attributed to problems with sexuality, the middle-aged with family problems, and the old with hard work and senility. These assumptions describe the normative Costa Rican life cycle of an early concern with sexuality and excesses, middle years of an expanding family and increasing responsibility, and an old age of suffering from hard work and neglect.

Differences in patient background such as the amount of time they had lived in San José also influence patient behavior. Patients from San José are more articulate with the doctor; those recently from rural areas more confused and hesitant. The long-term urban residents have used the pharmacies and emergency rooms more often before the observed consultation and the rural residents have used curers and private doctors. This pattern indicates local differences in access and beliefs which influence health care choice.

Within the Public Health and Social Security hospitals and clinics there are also teams of auxiliary medical personnel who work with the physicians to provide health care and social services. Nurses and social workers see patients in the hospital and visit patient homes to help families interpret medical recommendations and to supply physicians with information on patient home life and economic conditions. These extension services are an important link between the bureaucracy of the professional medical institution and the patient's family. Other medical personnel, such as aides, lab technicians, pharmacists, and a variety of hospital workers, provide professional sector medical services when they interpret medical advice or perform routine medical procedures. These medical workers also may use their medical skills outside of the hospitals and clinics by advertising their ability to give injections or suggest appropriate medical remedies. These practitioners are mentioned again both in the popular medical sector and at the end of the folk medical discussion, as some of these individuals practice more within an indigenous medical tradition than within the Western biomedical framework.

The professional medicine discussion has focused on patients and practitioners within the public sector of urban health care. There are no available statistics on the number of practicing private physicians, however, interviews with physicians suggest that most public sector practitioners also have some form of private consultation and Casas and Vargas report that "approximately one-third of all physicians have a private practice and fourteen percent of all medical consultations are made by private physicians" (1980: 268). Interview materials, ethnographic experiences, and brief observations of a few private consultations suggest that the private consultations differ from those in the public sector only in the degree of control the patient has in determining the course of interaction through direct payment. It is probably reasonable to assume that private patients are wealthier than public ones because of the higher fees, however, from the patient interviews there is evidence that even poorer patients consult physicians privately when advised to do so, or when they become disillusioned with the public institutions.

Popular Medicine: the Commercial Pharmaceutical Sector and Popular Religious Healing

Popular medicine in Costa Rica is based primarily on the use of home remedies, dietary control, and behavioral rules generated by the Galenic notions of hot and cold, as has been reported for most of Latin America. Preventive and remedial practices emphasize balance and equilibrium of intake and action for health (Low 1981). Popular medical practices also include religious petitions for health, the purchase of herbal substances in the marketplace, and family patterns of avoidance and magical influence.

In the urban environment of San José however, many of the popular remedies used at home and in self-care have been replaced by patent and prescription medicines purchased in local pharmacies and stores. Religious petitioning includes prayers to a saint but also to the sacralized image of a physician, Dr. Moreno Cañas. Thus, elements of the professional (Western biomedical) and folk (sacred folk healing) medical sectors are incorporated into the family and self-care domain that comprise popular medicine as a result of the urbanization process. I define health behavior that originates in the home as within the popular sector, even if the external characteristics of the behavior refer to or signify professional or folk practices.

Anne Ferguson in her study of Asuncíon, El Salvador, argues that "in Third World countries Western biomedical practitioners do not exercise the degree of control over the use of one of their major healing resources, prescription medications, that is characteristic of most Western developed countries. Instead, these products have become integrated into healing strategies of alternative medical practitioners, giving rise to a popular sector of medical care, here termed the commercial pharmaceutical sector" (1981: 105). In San José, Costa Rica, the utilization of pharmaceuticals is encouraged by the pharmacists and pharmacy staff and owners for commercial reasons, while the impetus for the purchase begins at home. Therefore, I consider the commercial pharmaceutical sector as part of popular health care.

Patients, searching for relief from a symptom, often start by asking at a *botica* or *farmacia* (pharmacy) for medicine or advice. As one pharmacist suggests, it takes less time, costs less money, and the pharmacist is a familiar figure concerned about the client's health problems and supported by the confidence of the neighborhood. Another pharmacist adds that the pharmacy provides an important public and social function. The pharmacist knows about medicine and its proper usage, and if he does not prescribe something, the client will go to someone who will. He believes that people are afraid to go to doctors because they think that the doctor will tell them that they have cancer or some feared disease.

Pharmacies may offer a preliminary diagnosis that will eliminate the symptoms. The pharmacist also may recommend a doctor for a secondary diagnosis and treatment when the symptoms persist and the patient reports that pharmaceutical treatment is unsuccessful. According to Costa Rican licensing laws pharmacists are limited in their clinical practice. Patients are required to present physician prescriptions for a large number of drugs and preparations. In actual practice, the role and expertise of the pharmacist is expanded to include important primary care treatment for a variety of minor ailments and problems. Prescriptions and patent medicine can be obtained "over the counter" by asking for the drug by name or pharmacological action.

There are basically two kinds of pharmacies in San José: the community or *barrio* pharmacy and the modern or commercial pharmacy. The community pharmacy has a traditional, stable clientele. The pharmacist gives personal advice and has direct contact with the client. Sales rely on responding directly to client needs and less on sundries and beauty items. To compete successfully, the pharmacist diagnoses illness and provides a treatment regime. The community pharmacist assures the citizens they are making the appropriate purchase and asks them to come again. The modern pharmacy, by comparison, is a commercial unit that specializes in the sale of patent medicines, relies heavily on sundry sales, and has a changing clientele. The pharmacist does not take the initiative or risk of giving advice or practicing any form of therapy. He does not carry many herbs nor prepare any of the traditional remedies commonly found in the community locale.

Historically, the community pharmacist established a therapeutic relationship that was the focus of primary care for the families of the barrio. In this sense, the pharmacist participated as an alternative health practitioner. With the proliferation of patent medicines and the development of a comprehensive health care delivery system, the small local pharmacies evolved into modern pharmacies and produced concomitant changes in the role of the pharmacist.

The following description of pharmacy use is presented from a lay patient point of view and therefore does not distinguish licensed (professional) from commercial practitioners. Both are called "pharmacists" and there is a blurring of distinctions between professional advice and the client's family health strategy. Thus, a Costa Rican informant comments on her own family's utilization of and relation with pharmacist Don Julio:

> I have heard of Don Julio ever since I was little. When any member of the family got sick my mother had always gone for Don Julio's advice. My mother hardly ever called the doctor for a home visit. We don't have a family doctor. In general, we are a very healthy family. My mother has always trusted Don Julio's judgment in her own health problems, and in all general health problems refers to him.
>
> When my mother wanted Don Julio to prescribe for me she would go to the pharmacy herself and tell him my symptoms and what was bothering me. Now when I need some advice, I ask the employee and he generally goes inside and asks Don Julio the question. I don't get to talk with Don Julio but he probably is able to see me through a panel that divides the public area and inside offices.

In an interview with Don Julio, he told of his first years of professional work when he was very active examining and diagnosing patients. After the war (World War II), doctors were very scarce and there was no Social Security. The neighborhood was more rural; now it has changed to higher income residents and his clientele is "middle-class." He commented that the pharmacy today cannot maintain itself with only the sale of medicines. In order for it to be a business, a pharmacy has to sell cosmetics, sundries, and other items. He thinks that the price of the medicine has psychological consequences that influence the efficacy of the drug. Don Julio went on to say that the preparation of herbs and natural medicines traditionally used has decreased; young doctors and pharmacists do not study these kinds of medicines. He studied their value and thinks that they work, even though he hardly uses them anymore. When recommending some medicine he always asks the client's age, symptoms, economic status, and medicines already taken.

Don Julio's comment on the necessity of selling cosmetics and other supplies was borne out by direct observation of the purchasing clients. Of 100 purchases made, 50% were of sundries, cosmetics, lotions, razors, and candies; 20% were patent medicines such as Vicks VapoRub, Alka-Seltzer, aspirin compounds (*Mejoral, Aspirina*); 10% were registered medicines sold without prescriptions; 6% vitamins; 4% herbal substances; and only 10% were doctor's prescriptions to be filled. In 8% of the purchases advice was sought as to the appropriate medicine or usage. From these observations, it appears that the professional medical role of the pharmacist in the city has contracted with the competition of free medicines from private doctors and prescription benefits at the Social Security and Public Health hospitals. Nonetheless, the popular medical role of the pharmacy has expanded; as one informant commented, she goes to the pharmacy most often when she is ill because she can purchase medicines for anything and can trust the pharmacist to advise her wisely if she does not know the remedy's name.

Other widely used forms of popular medicine are religious petition, oration, and promises to the patron saint of Costa Rica, the Virgen de Los Angeles. According to the classification of charismatic healing by Romano (1965), the Virgen de Los Angeles is a formal saint with international fame for her intercession to improve health and aid in curing disease. The use of religious petitions as a popular sector healing strategy is a common pattern found throughout predominantly Catholic countries and local populations.

Stories of the Virgen's miraculous cures are often dramatic, including economic as well as spiritual and physical health, and good fortune:

> Doña Juana was describing her 18 year old son's accident in which a truck hit him and left him in such a state that the doctor said that he would never walk again. The Doña said that she prayed to the Virgen de Los Angeles who performed the miracle and now he is fine. They therefore could use the insurance money from the accident to buy the house they now live in.

Testimonials to the Virgen's cures cover the walls of the Basilica de Nuestra Señora de Los Angeles in Cartago where her image first appeared to a young Indian girl in 1635 (Arrieta Q. 1960: 13). The handwritten statements often accompany small silver or gold replicas of the body part from which the petitioner suffered:

> Handwritten, under glass with a gold stomach attached: I thank with all my heart the Virgin of the Angels for the favor received, making this testimonial public. I had been suffering from ulcers of the stomach up until 39 days before they were going to give me an operation which could cut out half of my stomach. A new x-ray was taken and the doctor startled, said that there would be no necessity to operate as the ulcers had disappeared. This is a miracle of the Blessed Virgin of the Angels.
>
> Thank you my Mother. Your daughter, X, widow of Y.

Other testimonials thank the Virgen for helping them through an illness, an operation, or an accident:

Elaborate hand-lettered testimonial with photograph of a young girl:

The family X of the city of Granada, Nicaragua, infinitely thanks the little Virgin of the Angels, Queen of Cartago, Costa Rica, for the miracle bestowed on Miss X who was saved from a terrible typhoid fever that had her at the border of insanity.

Elaborate printing in gold block-letters with a color photograph of a boy with sunglasses:

I give infinite thanks to the Virgin of the Angels and to Jesus the Nazarene, for the bestowed miracle, the cure of an osteomyelitis of the foot of my son.

Handwritten, framed with a photograph:

I give thanks to the Virgin of the Angels for having saved the life of my brother when he fell from the fifth floor of a building.

Handwritten with before photograph and a large lock of hair:

I give thanks to the Queen of the Angels for the miracle of having returned my hair which fell out at the age of two years. And also gave me the miracle of speech.

Today I am five years old and I deposit my hair (to the Virgin) and also this photograph with much love to her and I recommended her devotion.

Petition to Dr. Moreno Cañas, the young doctor assassinated in 1938, is part of the cult practices and healing rituals in the popular medical sector. The majority of these health behaviors are performed by individuals in their homes. Dr. Moreno Cañas is reported to appear carrying a black doctor's bag and intervenes directly on the petitioner through operations, assisted by an accompanying nurse. In one interview, the informant reported that she had been in the hospital for her damaged spinal cord, but after the operation she was left partially paralyzed. She was very frightened, and the woman in the next bed told her to pray to Dr. Moreno Cañas. She prayed seriously and waited. During the night the Doctor came to her bed in a white coat accompanied by his nurse. He said he would have to operate and put her to sleep. The next morning she had regained control of her arm and leg; her doctor at the hospital stated that he could not understand what had happened, but thought it could be a change in treatment. The woman reports that Dr. Moreno Cañas continued to come every night for fifteen days; during each visit he checked and massaged her legs until she could walk and run again. She comments that he still works on the nerve in her leg, using a technique similar to the treatment the other hospital doctors are giving in physical therapy.

The interviews that focused on Dr. Moreno Cañas included beliefs and behaviors that also might be considered as professional medicine or sacred folk healing. Some interviewees had either seen him or known of his cures when he was alive. One woman had had an appointment with him for an appendectomy the day after he was killed. She said that he had come to her that night, the night of his death, and performed the operation. When she arrived at the office the next morning, the new doctor found that the operation was no longer necessary.

Other interviewees reported petitioning Dr. Moreno Cañas for minor problems, good fortune, and health. A supplication, such as the one below, is said and a glass of water and a candle, left out overnight; the doctor is said to visit the home and put medicine in the water which the supplicant then drinks in order to be cured.

> You, Doctor Moreno Cañas, the true source of light and wisdom, Grand Master, protector of all of whom in you believe. I ask of you with all my heart that you be the Doctor of our house and that you keep from me always the illness that I here state————, hoping once more to be protected by your great kindness.
>
> Here next to this Prayer I have left this glass of water and a candle so that with it you may illuminate your holy medicine, and ask of God that you never leave us unprotected in our suffering. Amen.
>
> I pray to God for us in our tribulations. (Say) An Our Father and an Ave Maria to ask God our Lord for the eternal glorification of our Great Doctor Moreno Cañas.

The belief in Dr. Moreno Cañas is widespread through the Meseta Central of Costa Rica. The sacralized image of a doctor performing healing functions incorporates elements of folk and professional medicine into lay health beliefs and practices expressed in popular religious healing.

Folk Medicine: Curers, Herbalists and Paramedical Practitioners

The literature of Costa Rica includes numerous references to the power and efficacy of the curer, spiritualist, and herbalist in the treatment of disease (Fallas 1973). The most complete study (60 interviewees) of these folk practitioners is of the town of San Miguel, a transitional suburb of San José, done by Dr. María Eugenia Bozzoli de Wille of the University of Costa Rica (1971: 1, 2). According to her, folk medicine is complementary to professional Western biomedicine and gains importance in cases where the professional medicine treatment is not succeeding, when the cost of the treatment is too expensive from the point of view of the patient or the family, or when there are no known scientific techniques or available facilities. The majority of the curing practices are of Hispanic origin; the use of candles, saints, the cemetery; the forms of divination; and the use of various plants of foreign origin were all introduced by the Europeans. The use of native plants constitutes the indigenous element, while the spiritualism aspects appear to have been an oriental influence employing Hindu or Buddhist vocabularies, (1971: 2: 78).

Practitioners reflected differences of age, sex, and background; about 60% supported themselves solely by curing, the remainder worked in a variety of paid occupations, using their practice to supplement their income (1971: 2:68). Patient socioeconomic characteristics were equally varied and reflect an urban clientele (Dobkin de Rios 1981). Of the sixty curers, ten were herbalists who did not cure witchcraft; nine were homeopaths who restricted their practice to empirical treatment of natural disease, and two were spirtualists who received all kinds of human ailments but did not cure or consult on the basis of spiritualism. The thirty-nine remaining curers treated disease, but also gave advice, medicines, and amulets against witchcraft and for good luck and travel; many divined by means of cards, reading palms, or glasses of water (Bozzoli de Wille 1971: 2: 71). Specific procedures for finding the origin of the evil or disease agent include communication by trance, dreams, or spiritual masters; and divination by cards, palms, intuition, oracles, or glasses of water. Healing procedures for preventing or curing evil include ritual cleaning of the body or home; keeping certain objects, amulets, medals, crosses, rosaries, or holy water nearby, either on the body or in the house; using medicines made by the curer or sold in a pharmacy; real or simulated surgery; and orations to folk saints or the devil in which certain numbers, usually three, seven or thirteen are important in the recitation or offerings (1971 1: 46–7).

Seven of the patients observed during the clinic consultations reported having tried a folk curer before coming to the medical clinic (Table II). One young man from the coastal region, reports that:

> ...all of his family had head illnesses. "*No creer ni dejar de creer*" (a saying meaning that one doesn't believe or give up believing). He thinks that some girlfriend could have done something to him. He says that his wife suffers because of him, he is irresponsible and not thinking things well. He thinks that it is witchcraft.

> He has been to several *curanderas* (curers) on the coast and in San José (mentions the name of one). He said that the curer gave him *baños* (bath of herbs) and elixirs which were useful. The curer didn't charge too much, only 15 colons ($1.80 in 1973). He thinks curers have as good a chance as anyone to cure him.

Another young man explains why he used a curer:

> He has a pain in his chest and left arm. Whenever he is worried this pain starts. His wife is very nervous, she sees and hears things. They went to a *curandera* for the attacks that she has. He took her to another city and to another Social Security doctor and the curer. He thinks it is witchcraft. He is recently married, and as soon as he was married his wife became pregnant and started acting bewitched. The child was premature and died. She is better now. He works on a farm as a sharecropper. He wants an x-ray, but the doctor says no, that the problem is in his head.
>
> He went to a curer in the city, but she was from the same village as he was (his wife's father had known someone who knew of this curer). It wasn't good to be from the same village as the curer so he went to another. The curer gave him a packet wrapped in tape and a small stone to work against the spell on his wife—there were two, one for the house and one to wear on his body. The curer also gave him colored liquid medicines for bathing and to take orally. Cost him 125 colons ($15.00) for one of the counter-spells. The doctor comments that it must be very good business.

A woman seen in the general medicine clinic relates that her illness has been previously treated, but wonders whether to continue the curer's instruction:

> She has had this itching and irritation of the skin for the past eight days. The doctor asks if she has eaten or taken any herbs. He gives her medicine and tells her that if it doesn't clear up he will send her to the skin specialist. And this pain of my side, the patient asks, "What does it mean?" "It means nothing," replies the doctor. Patient comments that for the last seven years her husband has been in bed and doesn't move because of a bewitching and a curse. She asks the doctor if she could take a medicine from the curer. The doctor jokes that she forget that medicine and take what he has ordered. She thinks that her husband is bewitched, and that maybe she is as well. She inquires again if she should take the medicine from the curer.

Home remedies (*remedios caseros*) were used by ten clinic patients either on their own initiative or on the recommendation of an herbalist, homeopath, or curer (Table II). One example is a man who had been receiving a successful treatment for a headache at Hospital Mexico:

> I've tried things at home—a slice of onion tied to the back of the head—that helped a lot but didn't cure me. A small towel soaked in hot black coffee alleviated the pain somewhat. I've been told, but haven't tried, a soup made of beef skull, and fish head soup.

Dr. Bozzoli de Wille reports that about seventy medications were mentioned by her informants for an entire spectrum of diseases including kidney problems, stomach ache, constipation, ovarian difficulties, waist pain, colic, obesity, headache, earache, nausea, liver problems, colds, skin eruptions, pneumatic pain, ulcer, sore throat, diarrhea, dandruff, intestinal parasites, asthma, colitis, tonsilitis, cough, and *nervios* (1971: 2: 67–8).

Herbalists are to be found selling dried preparations in some small local pharmacies, in stalls within the central market, and along the central plaza with hand trays of their remedies. A variety of medications are sold for such diverse ailments as a weak liver, impotency, tired blood, and general health maintenance. Most vendors profess an extensive knowledge of remedies and herbal treatments based on Galenic medical beliefs, while there are a number of herbal specialists whose businesses are devoted exclusively to female problems, children's illnesses, or selectively selling a quantity of one or two popular herbs. Clients visit these stalls either with specific home recipes to be filled or for direct consultation and prescription with the practitioner.

Other folk medicine practitioners include paramedical and non-medical advisors who do not practice as health specialists, but who offer services and limited consulting. These advisors are usually located within the neighborhood and work through personal and family networks. Some are isolated members of paramedical professionals such as midwives, chiropractors, homeopaths, and reflexologists. Other individuals are ex-nurses, aides, or hospital employees who provide such services as giving injections, explaining medical instructions, or offering home remedies (*remedios caseros*) to alleviate symptoms. The dividing line between popular and folk medicine becomes indistinguishable at this level of patient consultation.

These three medical sectors complete an overview of the Costa Rican health care system. The urban environment affords a diversity of practitioners and practices such that all these sectors and patient utilization patterns can be observed and codified.

Health Care Utilization

The medical sectors are used by urban patients during different illness episodes in various ways. The medical anthropological literature suggests that the afflicted individual responds to an illness based on the negotiated label or self-diagnosis (Murphy 1976), and that each label sets up an ordered hierarchy of resort to alternative curative practices (Romanucci Schwartz 1969); Nichter 1978, 1980). Therefore, the differential use of medical sector resources is primarily related to the nature of the disorder, the characteristics of the patients, and the features of the treatment systems (Colson 1971; Garrison 1977; Cosminsky and Scrimshaw 1980). The pattern of health care utilization describes the actual social organization of health care and reflects the cultural rules of appropriate health behavior for a particular illness category (Ugalde 1978). The heath-seeking process, the individually enacted response to perceived illness, can be conceptualized in terms of decisions about consultation, referral, treatment, and adherence (Chrisman 1977; Fabrega and Manning 1979; Fabrega and Zucker 1979; Young 1980, 1981).

The method selected to elicit illness strategies depended on hypothetical case questioning. My research assistant[1] and I used three common symptoms—headache, stomachache, and *nervios*—to elicit treatment choice in the order of use. *Nervios* is a cultural symptom related to family disturbance and social stress (Low 1981).

The interview sequence began with the question, "What would you do to alleviate a headache?" and a second phrase, "If that didn't alleviate it?" was repeated until the informant had no response or knew of no other treatment alternative. The responses for the three symptoms were similar, varying in the use of specific patent drugs. For instance, aspirin compounds or Alka-Seltzer were often cited for treatment of a headache, Donnatal or Milk of Magnesia for a stomachache, and Librium or Valium (common tranquilizers) for *nervios* and secondarily when other drugs did not bring relief. Patients reported widespread utilization of both professional and popular health care practitioners; folk practitioners were underrepresented because of the bias of the interview situation. We felt that interviewees were hesitant to discuss folk medical practices because of our association with the clinics. For this reason the data on folk practices are reported from ethnographic and secondary sources.

Based on the interviews, a number of utilization patterns for symptomatic treatment were used. For headache, five distinct patterns are detailed below.

LOCATION	TYPE OF TREATMENT
1) Pharmacy	Aspirin, Alka-Seltzer (Patent Medicine)
Public Health Clinic	Doctor (General Medicine)
Public Health	Specialist (Neurology)
Private Clinic	Specialist
2) Pharmacy	*Mejoral* (Brand of Aspirin)
Social Security Clinic	Doctor (General Medicine)
Social Security	Specialist (Psychosomatic Medicine)
3) Home	Herbal Remedy
Pharmacy	Aspirin, Alka-Seltzer (Patent Medicine)
Private Clinic	Doctor (General Medicine—"Couldn't wait for Social Security appointment")
Social Security Clinic	Doctor (General Medicine)
4) Pharmacy	Aspirin, Alka-Seltzer (Patent Medicine)
Home	Herbal Remedy
Social Security Clinic	Doctor (General Medicine)
Private Clinic	Doctor (General Medicine)
Social Security	Specialist (Neurology)
5) Home	Herbal Remedy
Pharmacy	Aspirin, Alka-Seltzer (Patent Medicine)
Pharmacy	Pharmicist (Prescription Medicine)
Social Security Clinic	Doctor (General Medicine)
Social Security	Specialist
Private Clinic	Doctor or Specialist

Common elements among these patterns lead to a generalized scheme for headache treatment:

LOCATION	TYPE OF TREATMENT
home	herbal remedy
pharmacy	Aspirin, Alka-Seltzer
clinic	doctor (from any system)
alternate clinic	doctor in another system and/or specialist in same system

Following the same process, the generalized patterns for stomachache and *nervios*, respectively, can also be summarized as:

LOCATION	**TYPE OF TREATMENT**
home	herbal remedy
pharmacy	Milk of Magnesia or Donnatal
clinic	doctor (from any system)
alternate clinic	doctor in another system and/or specialist in the same system

LOCATION	**TYPE OF TREATMENT**
home	herbal remedy (dandelion tea)
pharmacy	tranquilizers (Valium or Librium)
clinic	doctor (from any system)
speciality clinic	usually a psychiatric or psychosomatic specialist, although in some cases the patient went to many specialists for specific symptoms before entering a psychiatric clinic.
hospital	hospitalization usually at Chapui, the *asilo* (asylum)

It is inferred from the interviews that curer use would be part of step four in each sequence.

Teller (1972) produced similar results by surveying access to curative care in the Honduran city of San Pedro Sula during a two week period and calculating the rates of utilization. Of a total population of 1,000 persons, 311 became ill during the two week period, and of these 311, 99 did nothing, 103 used household remedies, 46 used private doctors, 49 used public doctors and 14 used curers (1972:89). The major difference is the use of public rather than private doctors in Costa Rica due to the increased availability of institutional physicians through Social Security clinics.

Woods (1977) in his analysis of alternative curing strategies in a Guatemalan town suggests that medical change moves from self-treatment to the use of minor resources such as the pharmacist or nurse to the use of major resources such as the physician and modern health care facilities. This order of curing strategies describes the hierarchy of resort and pattern of dual use in an urban setting as well as a change of treatment mode. The availability of multiple resources provides an environment in which a complex pattern of health care utilization may be seen as adaptive and health enhancing (Vayda 1974). Medical change as reported by Woods may be the description of how a complex urban health care system evolves. The studies of San José and San Pedro represent the most complex or developed organizational pattern of Latin American health care.

The choice of the initial clinic in San José is determined by occupation, whether the family has Social Security benefits, whether one clinic is believed to be more reliable, personable, or responsive to emergencies than the other alternatives. Each symptom has its own career with different outcomes. Early labeling of a symptom determines the direction and course of individual action. The cultural perceptions of illness etiology are also reflected in the health care choices.

There is variation in the pattern of treatment utilized for the different symptoms. Headache-stomachache-*nervios* form a continuum from the least to most complex hierarchy of resort. Headache has the simplest pattern including home remedy and physician-dependent therapies; stomachache treatment adds hospitalization; and *nervios* treatment further adds psychiatric consultation and a visit to, or hospitalization in, the Ministry of Public Health operated psychiatric hospital Chapui. The pattern produced by a combination of all three symptom patterns has four phases:

1. home treatment
2. pharmacy self-treatment and/or consultation
3. doctor consultation
4. alternate consultation

plus intervening additional steps as symptom requirements increase in complexity.

The addition of the specialist and psychiatric clinics is attributable to physician intervention and the professional referral system; the use of medicinal herbs, patent medicines, pharmacists, and the choice of the initial consultation relies primarily on the lay referral system (Friedson 1960). Treatment is controlled by the patient until he enters into a medical institution, at which time the direction of the treatment is influenced and modified by the physician. The degree of patient control is greater in the private physician fee-for-service system, and patients who wish to protect their health care decision-making role often use the private physician before entering into the larger medical institution. The patient attempts to keep health behavior within a familiar social context before entering the professional sector.

The medical hierarchy of resort replicates the basic social organization of Costa Rica, in which the family is the primary social arrangement and agent of social control, followed by the neighborhood, and finally the urban institutions and interrelated urban systems. At the family and neighborhood level, the patient is surrounded by familiar individuals and well-known, reliable remedies. As the patient moves to the institutional level, personal relationships are replaced by professional roles and statuses which limit personal prestige and control. These social organizational levels reach their greatest complexity in the urban environment, in that the diversity of local, neighborhood practitioners and the number of professional medical institutions increases, and patients are provided with maximum health care opportunities. This research confirms that the patient responds to the urban complexity by utilizing all levels of available care in any health seeking episode.

The description of San José health sectors, utilization patterns and hierarchies of resort predict health behavior at an individual level, in which the patient acts according to social and cultural rules of preferred health care. The individual, however, also acts in the context of social and cultural institutions. In San José, both the family and the principal medical institutions constrain and change individual health behavior from an ideal hierarchy of resort to family determined patterns of health care and institutionally controlled patterns of medical interaction.

CHAPTER III

FAMILY HEALTH CARE

The family in Costa Rica is the primary social institution that provides the basis of psychosocial identity. When a Costa Rican is asked for his name, he will respond with his *appellido* (his family name) rather than his personal name. A family is critical to economic maintenance as well as social support and single persons tend to live either at home or with another family (Low 1977). Individuals who break from their families or who are excluded by them, may express their social exclusion symbolically in the culturally appropriate symptom of *nervios* (Low 1981). Family, therefore, is necessary to health and individual well-being.

Research in the United States also has explored the importance of family context in health behavior and the treatment of illness (Parsons and Fox 1952; Mabry 1964). Studies have concluded that the role of the family in illness etiology may provide insights into the inclusion of family members in treatment (Minuchin, et. al. 1978). Family interaction is identified further as a source of psychosomatic disease process and illness control (Goldberg 1958; Titchener, et. al. 1960; Bursten 1964; Jackson and Yalom 1966). The family as a mediator of health care and as the major culture bearing unit which influences individual health behavior has been described for Mexican American families as they enter the United States health care systems (Clark 1970; Rubel 1966). Thus the patient may be described as being treated in the context of the family, with family members intimately involved in all health care decisions of the patient, including acceptance of diagnosis and treatment adherence. The family, not the patient, makes clinical decisions and directs health care seeking to such a degree that some authors suggest that the family be considered as the patient (Paul 1955).

This pattern of a strong family role in health care reoccurs throughout Latin America wherever the family retains its social structural dominance. Costa Rican families are no exception and influence patient health behavior and treatment.

The knowledge and values of family members determine patient explanatory models of disease process, illness and health-seeking behaviors (Kleinman 1980). These explanatory models reflect the cognitive structure of family expectations, explanations, and acceptable health behavior. Patient (family)-practitioner explanatory models often conflict, particularly in terms of disease etiology and appropriate treatment procedures; these conflicts impede health care delivery and patient compliance (Kleinman 1978; Locker and Dunt 1978).

The conflict between patient and practitioner explanatory models may account for the breakdown in communication during medical consultation. Studies of consumer satisfaction suggest that misunderstanding of expectations, clinical explanation, and treatment may lead to reports of patient dissatisfaction (Gray 1980). Young (1976) proposes that patient expectations are the major determinant of satisfaction. The examination of family case studies clarifies the relationship among patient expectations, clinical explanation, and patient satisfaction.

Family context also influences patient health care utilization patterns and the hierarchy of curative resort (Osterweis et. al. 1979). Patients begin their health seeking in the home, consulting family members, friends, and the local pharmacist before they enter medical institutions. Family-patient health behavior may incorporate a wide range of practitioners in diverse health care sectors or may focus on alternative practitioners within one medical setting. In Costa Rica, the health care strategies are hierarchical, in that one practitioner is utilized after another. Family values and socioeconomic status appear to monitor which of the health sectors will be used (Kurella 1979).

The relationship of family socioeconomic status and its impact on health sector utilization has not been fully explored. Kleinman states, with reference to Taiwan, that "only families in the upper middle-class treated all sickness episodes by resort to Western-style doctors, while only families who belonged to the lower-class treated all sickness episodes at home without resorting to professional or folk healer." (1980: 183). By contrast the urban Costa Rican hierarchy of resort is more integrated in that all social groups utilize the Western biomedical practitioners of the professional sector. However, the first conclusion, that upper middle income families use only the professional sector is confirmed in the present study. The importance of the relationship of socioeconomic status to health care utilization, however, may be in terms of the diversity of health care options that are perceived to be available to the particular family. The family cases from Costa Rica suggest that patient satisfaction is positively influenced by the number of health sectors that are utilized, and that these utilization patterns are related to socioeconomic status.

Differences in socioeconomic status in Costa Rica are reflected in lifestyle changes and identification with different values and social activities. The higher the family's socioeconomic position, the more likely they are to identify with North American cultural ideals and to perceive themselves as modern and up-to-date. The higher income Costa Ricans, therefore, prefer medical care that represents these values and use only Western, biomedically trained physicians.

However, this modern orientation does not affect all the behavior and values of the higher income class. Costa Rican scholars argue that a number of beliefs reflect cultural homogeneity and a lack of social differentiation (Rodríguez Vega 1953; Segovia 1951). For example, religious practices crosscut socioeconomic situations. Belief in the healing power of Dr. Moreno Cañas is held by individuals of all social statuses, although not necessarily acted upon by all. Education as a dominant theme in social mobility, socialization of children, economic opportunity and achievement is respected by all socioeconomic groups. Further, ideals concerning sex role segregation, family solidarity, and the importance of family continuity are stressed in all families.

Worldview and the scope of social activities, however, varies with socioeconomic status. Professional families visit the United States, utilize a wide range of stores and locations for shopping and services, and demonstrate an extensive knowledge of political and legal systems. Middle income and upwardly mobile families use the urban environment extensively and visit the countryside, but the scope of their contacts and activities is confined to national limits. In lower income families the social world and perceived opportunity are radically narrowed; social life is restricted to personal contacts, local employment, family and neighborhood interaction. The poorest families live in the most circumscribed world where the extent of a woman's participation outside the home is her visit to the local health clinic.

The Family Interviews

The following description and analysis of the influence of family context on health behavior in Costa Rica is based on nine family cases. The patients and their families, articulate about their problems and perceptions, were viewed as key informants in the identification of the patterns of family influence on health behavior in Costa Rica.

The patients selected were in some ways similar to other observed patients: their symptoms were a mixture of somatic and psychological complaints and about a third of them had *nervios* (Low 1981); their clinical explanations ranged from family and economic worries to folk notions of *alimento* (food or nourishment) and brain weakness, and their requests for treatment included medications, examinations, and explanation of their illness. But because of the way the patients were chosen they differ from the clinic population. The selected patients are all female, ranging in age from twenty-five to sixty-five, and four of the nine women are divorced or single. The emphasis in the analysis is on the relationship of variables within each family rather than on the family data as a sample.

Each patient was interviewed with her family at home by a male research assistant and myself. A structured interview schedule[2] was used to guide the order of questions and to insure that the same questions were asked in each home. The families varied in their responses such that some interviews took five to six hours to complete, while others were completed over many days. In many cases each member of a family wanted to respond to each question individually; each such response was recorded separately. These interviews are summarized in the family cases.

Patient expectations, clinical explanations, and satisfactions were collected by posing a series of questions to the patient before and after medical consultation. Interviews were done in the waiting room of the outpatient clinics of the Social Security and Public Health hospitals. The results of these interviews are presented after the family description in each of the nine family cases. In this way the reader can compare the family context and health care utilization with the patient's own report of expectation, clinical explanation and satisfaction.

Family Case Studies

Family 1

The informant lives with her parents in a traditional large wood frame house in the center section of the city. The house is embellished with Victorian wood trim, an iron gate, and hand-painted Spanish tile floors. The decor is conservative and simple, with old silk-covered furniture and elegant wallpaper. The informant has her own suite within the house and drives her own car. A maid answers the door and sees us in.

The household is composed of the informant's mother, father, and her infant. Her sisters, who live close by, are seen daily. A full-time *empleada* (domestic) cares for the ailing mother and a second domestic helps with housework and watches the baby.

The informant is a Spanish professor who attends night courses to complete a graduate degree. She earns US $350 (1973) per month with which she supports her child. Although her income would allow her to support herself independently, she prefers to remain with her family. Her father is an established businessman and farmer; his income covers all household expenses.

The family has always lived in the same neighborhood and "knows everyone." The informant feels that living alone away from home and neighborhood would be impossible. She prefers to study rather than work and believes that a woman with a child should stay at home and not leave the child with an *empleada.* Affection and a stable home are the most important aspects in a child's life. Both parents should discipline the child. She explained that the father of her child was waiting for a divorce so she had had a "contract marriage" drawn up by a lawyer, giving the child his father's surname. She does not want to marry or even have a boyfriend now. This arrangement is culturally unusual and may reflect a more complex personal situation.

The informant shops once a week with her mother. She attends classes at the University in the evenings and goes on outings every weekend with her child and best friend. She says that she tells her best friend everything and that they are very close.

Her health is generally good, though her child has been bothered by *nervios.* The informant says that she suffers most from depression. Her family uses the Social Security specialty clinics, or a private doctor if the problem is urgent.

Patient interview before and after the medical consultation

Patient complaint: I feel depressed, but not like

before. I am afraid to go out alone, and still feel persecuted.

Patient expectation: The doctor and I are good friends. I come here as though it were a confession; confidence in the doctor is important

Patient explanation of her illness: Dissatisfaction with job and life. I can not tell you where the problem came from... external (vague description).

Patient satisfaction: Did not like the consultation with the doctor. I was not talking so he gave me more medicine.

Family 2

The house is located in a new subdivision of San José, surrounded by other large, modern stucco homes. It is decorated with contemporary matching furniture, all possible appliances, a terrazzo floor and a snack bar where the children can eat and watch television. A smart young *empleada* answers the door and calls the "mistress of the house."

The household consists of the informant, her husband, their ten year old son, and twelve year old daughter. The informant's sister, who works as a consultant for the government advising workers, stays with them every week-end. They have a live-in *empleada* who cares for the house and does some cooking. The husband works for a large government institute earning almost U.S. $1,000 (1973) per month. The wife remains in the home watching the children and performing small domestic tasks. Although parts of their extended families are scattered throughout the country and the United States, both of their mothers are still nearby and they visit them weekly. The informant was previously married to a employee of a large cacao company and had lived in the coastal region. She had come from a poor family and has now married a man socially more prestigious than her own family. Her son by her first marriage is a doctor; he married a girl who the mother disapproves of and now lives and practices medicine in an outlying provincial region of Costa Rica. They do not see the son except to pick up the grandchild.

The informant likes her neighborhood and feels very comfortable with the neighbors. She does not think that women with children should work, nor does her husband. It is important to her that all her neighbors are just like her; she feels very safe knowing that she is surrounded by families with similar concerns.

She believes that health and education are the two most important things in bringing up children and that only the father should discipline them. She manages the household and shopping, and goes to the American style supermarket once a week. They read, travel, go to parties, and to the beach for recreation. They have numerous acquaintances and friends, but the wife has no best friend; she does not like to be that close to people, she just likes to talk with them.

In the past few years, the health of the wife has been poor. She most often suffers from colitis and attacks of *nervios*. The family uses the pharmacy or friends of the informant's son if it is a "light" illness, and the Social Security hospital if "serious." She has also consulted a homeopath, an osteopath, and a curer (*curandera*) during various illness episodes. She has "seen" Dr. Moreno Cañas and recounts being cured by him many times (Low 1982).

Patient interview before and after the medical consultation

Patient complaint: Daughter has headaches and inflamed tonsils; son has come for a check-up.

Patient expectation: X-rays for the daughter, and the doctor should just see the son.

Patient explanation of daughter's illness: Headaches are from television and school or from growing. Son has nothing wrong.

Patient satisfaction: "Went well, the doctor is very attentive; he asked about things I had forgotten about. The doctor agreed about the x-rays, gave anti-allergy pills, examined both children and ordered exams of urine and blood. I am very happy because he gave my daughter the x-ray exams."

Family 3

The traffic and movement of people in this house never seems to stop. The house is a Spanish colonial, stucco and tile building located in an old established neighborhood. The interior is large and spacious, with an assortment of furnishings and antiques; there are chickens, birds, cats, and dogs in the yard. The sister answered the door.

The household is an extended family made up of the infomant, her mother and father, two brothers, and one sister. One of the brothers is married with two children who also live in the house, and the sister has a young son. Female solidarity is strong with much teasing, joking, and friendly interaction between the mother and sister-in-law, and the sister-in-law and the informant. The father is a businessman. The two brothers work for governmental agencies, and both sisters are preparing for professional careers in medicine and literature. The total income from all members is about US $500 (1973) per month plus commissions. The other married brother and his wife visit daily and live only four blocks away. The family pays rent on this house, but has an option to buy, and would like to pay off the house or build another one with an apartment to rent.

The mother grew up in an upper class household in another city. She likes to be out of the house, and thinks that women should work outside the home, although her husband does not agree. This attitude has influenced the informant's life goals; she is now pursuing a degree at the University of Costa Rica. According to the informant, education and religion are the most important ingredients of a child's upbringing.

The activities of the generations is clearly differentiated. The mother shops daily for perishables, and weekly for dry goods. Her recreation is limited to watching television, visiting the grandmother, or going to the country only twice a year. The informant, however, often goes to the movies, parties, and dances, and participates in all aspects of urban San José life. She is enrolled at the University and works for her father part time. These activities have broadened her experience and life goals. As a family they have acquaintances, but no close friends. Gatherings at home are made up of the mother's sisters and brother from a nearby city. The informant has friends and acquaintances at the University, but they do not visit her at home.

Her health and the health of the family is good. Her father suffers most from *nervios*, the informant has ulcers and colitis, and her mother has had pain from her rheumatic shoulder. The family goes to a private doctor at Hospital San Juan de Dios for medical treatment.

Patient interview before and after the medical consultation

Patient complaint: Last Sunday she ate a *biscocho* (hard cookie) and had an "epileptic fit," lost consciousness and vomited. (This is the patient's description. Costa Ricans often refer to *descomposiciones*, or fainting spells, as part of their cultural repertoire of illness. This reporting may be a variation of the cultural symptom).

Patient expectation: Results of the x-rays. "He is going to tell me today where the attack came from and why I had such an episode. He will give me pills for my nerves."

Patient explanation of her illness: It's psychological. I assume it came from nerves. Perhaps it was caused by my exams at school.

Patient satisfation: It only went relatively well. "He says the headaches are from my eyes so they will send me to an eye doctor to see about that. The tests were negative. He told me nothing, that it was just nerves."

Family 4

It is a long and narrow wooden home, immaculate, with fabric upholstered sofa and chairs. The front room doubles as a bedroom for the informant. She lives alone in this house with her two sons and *empleada*; her mother lives a few houses away. She answered her own door.

The informant is a divorced school teacher. Her ex-husband is a technician who does not send money regularly. All together her income is about US $200 (1973) per month, but her mother helps, and they share food and cooking at times. She does not like the house or the neighborhood but rented it to be close to her mother. She would like her own house and is studying to obtain a graduate degree which will increase her salary and teaching possibilities. She likes to work, but feels that a woman with children should not have to. She tries to provide the most important thing, affection, to her children. She says that she is a very caring parent. Since she works, the maid does the shopping daily in the central market.

She likes to go to the country, and often goes with her children and friends from work. There is a group of divorced women who often spend time together and provide one another with recreational companionship and emotional support. She does not have people to the house and does not spend time with the neighbors. She says that she is part of the "middle class." She recognizes that she would like a better life, but as a divorced woman, she is culturally sanctioned and feels at a disadvantage. She has had to work very hard to maintain her own home without an extended family or a husband.

She suffers from asthma, colitis, and *nervios*. The family goes to a private doctor for primary care, but uses the Social Security clinic for specialists and hospitalization. A long time ago she tried calling on Dr. Moreno Cañas, but felt so strange that she has not done so again.

Patient interview before and after the medical consultation

Patient complaint: Headache, throat problem, frigidity, eyes hurt, crying.

Patient expectation: "A very deep analysis. I have faith the doctor can help. If physical then it's easy, he will just inject some *alimento* (nourishment). If psychological, then he will have to look out for the root of the problem. I want advice, a cleaning out of the brain. I want him to study my case." (The relationship of brain and alimento is through a folk illness category "brainache". Brainache is thought of as a syndrome of *debilidad del cerebro,* debility of the brain, caused by a lack of *alimento,* vitamins or healthy food (Low 1981). There is both a somatic and psychological meaning to these concepts, and I believe she is using that ambiguity in her expectation.)

Patient explanation of her illness: "I think my nerves wear out my body. It could be because of frigidity. I think that the frigidity perhaps is because of something done to me when we were first married. Maybe it was the honeymoon thing or my husband's inexperience." (Here, the informant is referring to her unhappy, broken marriage. Frigidity implies again both an emotional and sexual meaning.)

Patient satisfaction: "He gave me some pills for my headache. I don't like them (pills) and don't take them anyway. The nurse had to explain the medication. It didn't go well."

Family 5

The informant lives in an extended family household that occupies two contiguous wooden houses, both long and narrow, facing along the street. There is constant activity of ironing, washing, cleaning going on by the women of the house as other family members come and go, calling greetings and questions, not waiting for responses. The informant had permission to leave work early for the interview and invited all family members, who were in either house, to join in with information and advice. Everyone tried to speak at once, so much so that the research assistant and I split the group, each interviewing half, at the same time.

The informant is a young woman who lives with her infant son and her two unmarried sisters in the house of her parents. Her married brother and his family live next door and her other six brothers and sisters all live close by in the same community. The "family," as defined by the informant's mother, includes her ten children, her 42 grandchildren and the six great-grandchildren. The parental home is the center of all activities where everyone gathers at least once daily. Daughters-in-laws are teased and actively participate in the friendly banter and horseplay of the household.

The informant works as a clerk in a hardware store in the center of San José. The father of her child also had worked there, but left; he will not recognize the child nor help with the expenses. She does not earn very much, about US $75–100 (1973) per month, but that money is just for her child and their personal expenses. All the daughters contribute some amount to the running of the house, but the house is owned by the family, so no rent is paid. The father works locally and the other sisters work in large department stores where they can earn better wages. The informant lives a restricted life. Her mother does not allow her to go out alone or to go even to the market. She watches television for entertainment. She is happy working and feels that sometimes it is necessary for a woman to work even when she has a child.

The most important parts of a child's upbringing are his education, food, and cleanliness. Her mother and father discipline her child which causes problems and friction when her instructions conflict with her parents' rules. She does not have any friends but does know some of the people she works with. Basically, her life is filled with her family and their activities. She would like a life of her own because of family conflict over the discipline of her child, but says that it would be impossible because she would have no way to support herself alone.

She has had a series of minor illnesses, the major complaint being a problem with her tonsils. She has been to a private doctor, a homeopath, the Social Security clinic, and to curers (*curanderos*). She prays to the Virgen de Los Angeles for better health. Her mother is a devotee of Dr. Moreno Cañas and consults a spiritualist in an attempt to cure her own *nervios* and stomach distress.

Patient interview before and after the medical consultation

Patient complaint: Back (*columna*) hurts, also has bad tonsils and a bit of arthritis.

Patient expectation: An injection to alleviate the pain; an injection of *espasmo cibalgina*. "The pains you can not get rid of with just anything. I want to know what it is before I get the medicine. Here they give the same medicine for different pains. I am going to ask for what I want. Also want an x-ray." (The drug mentioned is a commonly known prescription pain reliever.)

Patient explanation of pain: Hurt is a result of a fall.

Patient satisfaction: "The doctor gave me an urgent order for an x-ray and medication. Now I will find out what is wrong. I received good treatment. I have no complaints."

Family 6

The house is one-half of a duplex, made of wood, quite small, and in poor repair. The husband of the informant is presently building another modern cement house for his son down the street, and they say that when they have the money he will build his family another house as well. They live on the edge of the city in what was an old town center. The house is poorly furnished with plastic covered chairs and broken wood floors; beds cover most of the space, and the walls are covered in photographs, magazine clippings, diplomas and certificates of classes completed. The kitchen is the activity center of the house, full of medicinal plants and herbs; wooden benches, stools and tables. Here the family congregated to drink coffee and talk.

The family consists of the husband and the informant, their two daughters, a child of the first daughter, the child and the husband of the second daughter and the son of a daughter who lives in another barrio. The last daughter runs a bar and has left her son in her mother's house because she does not have time to care for him. The three other daughters, sons-in-law and their children all live a block away. The only living parent has remained in the countryside, and the family goes to see him every two weeks.

The wife likes to work and always has, but can not now because she is frequently sick. Her husband is a construction worker who builds houses and other buildings earning about US $100 (1973) per month. One of the daughters helps by working in a factory, and the son-in-law drives a van. The total income for the extended family household is about US $200 (1973) per month. They have no friends and only family comes to the house. Friendships are thought only to cause problems. They rarely go out (four times in thirty-one years) and watch little television; instead the family listens to the radio during their work. The most important parts of a child's upbringing are his cleanliness and food.

The mother and daughter shop daily at the central market. They take the long bus ride downtown to save the expense of buying at high local prices. The wife says that they are *gente humilde* (humble people) and must defer to the rich.

The entire family has had a long series of illnesses. The wife has chronic gastritis, *derrames* (strokes), fainting spells, and other psychosomatic complaints. Her daughters have had a series of complaints; ovarian problems, tonsilitis, and hepatitis. One daughter seems to have "mental" problems, and she has sought help through religious prayer to stabilize her family life through focusing on the relearning of sex roles and appropriate behavior. The family was not specific about the kind to mental illness, but commented that she acted strangely. The family usually goes to the Social Security clinic or may go to San Juan de Dios. The informant is a firm believer in Dr. Moreno Cañas and once saw his hand come to cure her. She also uses a pharmacist and homeopath to treat disorders. She has a large garden of medicinal herbs in her backyard which she uses to treat herself and her extended family.

Patient interview before and after the medical consultation

Patient complaint: Chronic gastitis.

Patient expectation: The doctor always examines me and gives me medicine.

Patient explanation of illness: "Caused by a certain debility from not eating, lack of *alimento* that causes the intestine to dry out." (*Alimento* refers to healthy or nourishing food in this context.)

Patient satisfaction: "It went well. The doctor examined me and found me better. He gave me medicine. I will continue my treatment with this doctor. With him I have gained two and one-half pounds. The doctor explained well; I understood well. The doctor is a very good doctor with me."

Family 7

The informant lives in a one room section of a low narrow building with a shared washing area, toilet, and shower. The room itself is quite small, filled with a double bed, a two-burner stove, table and chairs. There is a refrigerator, television, and radio. The room is carefully decorated and has a bar with matching equipment in a corner which was pointed out as very valuable. The informant is dressed up for the interview and sees us alone.

In this room live the informant and her "boyfriend". The informant has a grown son who is mentally retarded and remains in the parental home with her father and stepmother. She sees her son and father every two weeks, otherwise she does not see any family. She would like her son with her, but her boyfriend would not like it. He works at a bar and fights bouts of alcoholism. She does not work regularly but sometimes sells things and runs a raffle among local residents. They get along with most of their neighbors and have friends over to drink.

She feels that it is good to work. Her boyfriend understands that she likes to work and to have pretty things, although he does not really like her out of the house. She only shops and cooks for herself as he eats at the bar. She likes to dance and to go out. She listens to the radio all day long, but still she is very bored. Before she used to work as a dancer, and then she really enjoyed life. They were happy then, but now there are too many problems. She thinks that education and affection are very important for a child. She feels she is middle class and aspires to having nice things.

Basically she uses the pharmacy and the Public Health hospital for health care. The public hospitals also took care of her son for many years. She has a chronic case of *nervios* for which her father finally took her to Chapui to be treated. There she received some consulting and medication which have helped. She took her son to a curer many years ago, but it did not help as she does not have enough faith. She has not returned.

Patient interview before and after the medical consultation

Patient complaint: Has headaches and nerves.

Patient expectation: Pills and explanation of her illness.

Patient explanation of complaint: "came from boyfriend who drinks a lot. He threatens her. Also family worries." She does not get along well with her stepmother.

Patient satisfaction: "The doctor prescribed something and ordered another appointment. The doctor was pleasant. He appeared to understand the family problems, but he didn't explain. I'm not sure about the pills, he didn't tell me about them. I might come back if I don't get better—but if at all better would rather not return."

Family 8

The house is built of rough, unfinished wood, in typical Costa Rican country style. A car top spans the drainage ditch to enter the door. The neighborhood appears rural, with a semi-paved road, and no bus service. Women are washing clothes outside, in front of their homes; the chickens, ducks, and other animals run freely about the yard. The interior of the house is also rough wood, with wooden stools and a table with a plastic cover. Partitions divide up the rest of the house. The cold wind is blowing through the doors and plastic covered windows. The room is quite bare, filled only with a radio, cots, umbrellas, benches.

The informant lives with her husband, three children, and her brother. Her parents live next door, and she visits with her mother and sister daily, but does not speak with her father because they fight whenever he drinks. Her husband is a *peon* (farmhand) and makes about US $60–75 (1973) per month. Her brother is looking for work but so far has found nothing. Her mother sends food over to the brother and also cleans his clothes. They are paying off the lot the house is on and they have plans to rebuild the house. She likes the neighbors although she says that she does not visit with them. She has no friends and only says hello to people when they pass. She would like to work but right now she can not. She thinks that one must find a trustworthy person to leave one's children with and that it is important to supplement the husband's income. The husband would not approve unless she worked in the same place as he did.

Recreation is usually a walk in a pasture with the children. She listens to the radio all day long but does not have a television. For them problems are economic. They say they are poor and only education can change that.

The family is always sick. She has colds, asthma, and uterine problems. Both she and her mother suffer from *nervios*. For illnesses, they go either to the pharmacy or to the local Social Security clinic. She has always used a homeopath, a woman who gives injections, and prayers to San Martin de Porres and La Reina (Virgen) de Los Angeles.

Patient interview before and after medical consultation

Patient complaint: Behavioral disorder of her son. He is very restless at bedtime.

Patient expectation: "Sympathy, a way of treatment. Pills. The doctors, they show you hope."

Patient explanation of her son's illness: From her family; they are also nervous; it is heredity and environment.

Patient satisfaction: "I feel fine and will continue with medicine, cure with pills. The way the doctor dealt with us agreed with me. He gives you a manner with which you can express yourself. Doctor put explanation of medicine on the box (container of medicine) and gave us new appointments. Eddie liked the treatment of the doctor. They conversed a lot. I can now go home tranquil. The doctor understood. He gave me counsel about my marriage and how to treat Eddie."

Family 9

The home of the informant and her family is an old *peon's* house on what remains of a coffee plantation in the process of becoming a subdivision. A rotting wooden crossing over the ditch at the roadside leads down to the rundown, unmaintained wooden structure. Another room had been added to the house to accomodate the son's family when he married. During most of the interview there was a constant movement of family members—the married son's children would run in, ask for cookies, and jump on the bed.

The household includes the informant and her husband, who have been married for thirty years, their three sons and two daughters, the wife of one of the sons and their three children. The husband works on the farm and makes about US $50 (1973) per month. One son works at a press, another as a helper in a store, and the third cannot find work. All together the family probably brings in $150 (1973) per month. The entire family lives together; no other relatives were mentioned except a brother who is seen once a year. They do not visit their neighbors (the neighborhood is broken up by the subdivision) and feel that everyone should stay in his own house. They would like to buy their own lot there before all the land is subdivided. The informant says that she has no friends. She stays home and watches television or reads the Bible. She goes out only to visit the medical clinic.

The most important things in bringing up children are to feed them well, keep them clean and protect them from danger. Their ideal would be to have a farm with animals, but feel that probably buying a lot would be more within their financial means.

Although the informant said that her health was good, the family medical record indicates that she has been ill and hospitalized many times, particularly for mental illness, as she was hospitalized at Chapui. She has suffered from *nervios* and colitis, as well as high blood pressure and difficult childbirth. Her children also complain of *nervios*, bronchitis, and a series of congenital problems such as crossed eyes, brain damage, and learning disabilities. The family uses the Social Security system and the Public Health clinics for their health care as well as a number of home remedies, and pharmacist and folk curer consultations.

Patient interview before and after the medical consultation

Patient complaint: Bad comprehension, fears (*susto*).

Patient expectation: "The doctor will ask questions about how I feel. He will tell me how to carry on at home. He will give me capsules and vitamins for my brain."

Patient explanation of her illness: Lack of *alimento* for her brain.

Patient satisfaction: "Went very well. Medicine was prescribed and the doctor explained. I didn't know the doctor, but he seemed to be a very good specialist."

Family Context and Variables of Patient Satisfaction

The relationship of family context to patient satisfaction reflected in these nine cases is based on the three variables of: 1) patient expectation, 2) explanation and 3) health care section utilization. These three variables emerge as important in distinguishing patients 1, 3, 4, and 7, who expressed some form of dissatisfaction with the consultation, from patients 2, 5, 6, 8 and 9, who reported greater satisfaction with their medical encounter. The data derived from the patient and family cases presented in Table IV illustrate this relationship.

The satisfied patients have expectations such as pills, injections, physical examinations, and x-rays, which the doctor can and does fulfill. Some satisfied patients want to know what their illness is, or to be asked questions and given advice, but these requests for an information exchange do not seem to indicate an underlying desire for a life change or psychological readjustment, which is expressed in the expectations of dissatisfied patients. Most satisfied patients directly articulate their expectations, without recourse to alternating physical and psychological expectations based on differential diagnosis (see case 4). In all cases the expectations of satisfied patients are met during the consultation.

The dissatisfied patients' expectations, however, are not fulfilled. Their requests tend to be more psychological than physical, requiring greater explanation and longer term solutions not provided by the physician's services in a single consultation.

Patient expectations and satisfaction in terms of the practical, social, and symbolic or existential meaning of the healing interaction have been discussed by Allan Young (1976). The practical level of medical evaluation is determined by whether the

Table IV
Family Variables and Patient Satisfaction

Family Patient	*Variables*			*Patient*	
	Expectation	*Explanation of Illness*	*Health Sector Utilization*	*Satisfied*	*Dissatisfied*
1	confession, confidence	dissatisfaction with job and life, problem is external	professional		X
2	x-rays, examination	from television, school, growing	professional, popular, and folk	X	
3	results of x-rays, where attack from and why	psychological, nerves	professional (in the past used other sectors)		X "relatively well"*
4	deep analysis, advice, a cleaning out of the brain, study my case	nerves, frigidity	professional		X

5	injection, x-ray, to know what it is	hurt as a result of fall	professional, popular, and folk	X	
6	examination, medication	debility from not eating, lack of *alimento*	professional, popular, and folk	X	
7	pills, explanation of illness	from boyfriend, family worries	professional (in the past used other sector)		X "rather not return"*
8	sympathy, treatment, pills	from family, heredity, and environment	professional, popular, and folk	X	
9	asked questions, given advice and capsules	lack of *alimento*	professional, popular, and folk	X	

* The exact phrase has been included to indicate that in these two cases the dissatisfaction was not as strong as in cases 1 and 4.

treatment "works", i.e. what the patient expects to happen in fact does. The social level refers to the quality of the interaction between healer and the patient, and the symbolic or existential level acknowledges the ontological importance of health and healing in the definition of human action and experience.

The expectation data from the family cases can be understood in terms of these levels. Satisfaction is reported when the consultation "works" by fulfilling the patients' practical expectations; when the physician confirms their social relationship by performing the expected medical ritual; and when the physican affirms the patients' existence by resolving the health crisis through proper treatment. The patients who express diffuse and psychological expectations do not experience healing at these three levels. The patient who wants a deep analysis (case 4), does not get one in a five minute consultation, nor does the physician confirm his relationship with her or resolve her discomfort because his treatment options are limited.

Patient explanations of illness further differentiate the psychological and emotional etiologies of dissatisfied patients from the biophysical and environmental etiologies of satisfied patients. Patient explanations of illness etiology and treatment expectations overlap to form patient explanatory models of specific illness events. These models, when complete, include explanations of etiology, time and onset of symptoms, pathophysiology, course of sickness, and treatment (Kleinman 1980: 105). Practitioner explanatory models often conflict with those of patients and their families; when this occurs, the patient may feel dissatisfied and frustrated that the physician doesn't understand his case. In the family cases, it appears that the explanatory models of the dissatisfied patients report psychological etiologies for their illnesses and expect some kind of emotional or analytical response to their problems. The physician's treatment in these cases was to give medicines, based on his own explanatory model and interpretation of the situation. The treatment is incongruent with the patient's explanatory model and, therefore, the patient feels dissatisfied.

Explanatory models can differ in more than etiology. Case 3 presents evidence that the doctor and patient in fact agree on nerves as the etiology of her problem. The source of dissatisfaction is that the doctor told her nothing, while the expectation was that he would tell her where the problem came from and why. In this case, then, even though the physician's and the patient's explanations are the same, their assumptions of appropriate treatment are different and result in patient dissatisfaction. In other words, their explanatory models, which include beliefs about etiology and treatment, were not compatible.

The third variable, family health care utilization, ties the family pattern of health-seeking behavior to the individual outcome of patient satisfaction. Families of satisfied patients use all three health sectors—professional, popular, and folk—for medical treatment and consultation. Families of dissatisfied patients, however, use only the professional sector, usually a private doctor or the clinics of major medical institutions. In two cases, families 3 and 7, the patients utilize the professional sector but report having used another sector in the past. Both patients state that they no longer believe in or use the previous models of health care. These two patients also report dissatisfaction in a milder verbal form than patients 1 and 4. Their responses conform on the first two variables, patient expectation and explanation with the other dissatisfied patients, but on the utilization variable, they are in an intermediate position. Their degree of dissatisfaction appears less defined than the other patients, possibly because of their distinctive use of health care. The sensitivity of the dissatisfaction indicator suggests that the three variables may influence patient reactions independently.

The health care utilization variable also is explained by family socioeconomic status. The family cases suggest that increased education and income restricts rather than expands health care options. That is not to say that wealthier patients do not see a larger number of practitioners. Kleinman has confirmed the "well-documented cross-cultural patterns in which greater utilization of health care services correlate with higher socioeconomic status when such services operate on a fee-for-service basis" (1980: 183–4). However, the lower socioeconomic status patients in the family sample utilize a greater number of health care sectors. Differences in family lifestyle and medical beliefs correspond to the differences in health behavior.

The dissatisfied patients 1, 3 and 4 (excluding patient 7) are all professionals, with varying degrees of family mobility and economic support. Their degree of education is reflected in a medical orientation that narrowly defines health care in terms of the professional sector and Western biomedicine. Their complaints, however, are generalized and expressed in non-biomedical terms. Their restricted health care options do not correspond to their psychological and emotional definition of illness; the patient-physician encounter is limited in time and interview content, and is therefore perceived as unsatisfactory. The families of lower socioeconomic status (also including patient 2 in which the informant has recently married into a family of substantially higher status) utilize a broader range of health care practitioners including spiritualists, homeopaths, pharmacists, herbalists, and curers. Their understanding of cure and degree of reported satisfaction relies less on the limited psychological ability of the medical practitioner because of a large repertoire of available health behavior.

The dissatisfied patient in family 1 wanted to make a confession and have confidence in her doctor, expectations which could be fulfilled more easily in a religious healing context. However, her expressed modern and affluent attitudes are not compatible with religious healing as a health care alternative. The dissatisfied patients in families 3 and 4 reflect a similar conflict. Both patients want an explanation of "why" a set of disturbing symptoms had occurred. Their expectations are a mixture of moral, metaphysical, and practical requests and the treatment of symptoms is inadequate to satisfy the non-clinical needs. These expectations, however, could have been fulfilled by a folk healer or spiritualist who might have provided them with the answer to the "why" of their illnesses. The use of multiple therapies as a means to health care satisfaction is an important variable to consider in evaluating family strategies of health-seeking behavior.

The family context as reflected in the family interview may further influence individual health behavior through the value orientation elicited by the question on the most important aspects of childrearing. Of all the family variables analyzed—household composition, socializing patterns, attitudes towards women's work—childrearing ideals most clearly distinguish satisfied and dissatisfied patients. The informants responded in basically two ways: 1) a traditional response included food, cleanliness, health, and education as the most important and 2) a less traditional, more modern response included affection, religion, and a stable home as the more important ingredients, often combined with education. This split in response pattern can be attributed to a dominant value placed on child well-being (*bien estar*) or health, which is culturally based on proper food, cleanliness, and behavior—behavior being judged by proper conduct acquired through education. Psychological ideals of affection, religion, and a stable home were traditionally regarded as givens, not qualities that must be developed or encouraged. Only in the more modern families are these values presented as the necessary ingredients of childrearing. Their changing lifestyles and acceptance of North American cultural patterns either has modified their perceptions of what is important and culturally required or has made the delivery of these traditional ideals more problematic. This difference in value orientation, the traditional to modern shift, also differentiates medical consultation satisfaction, reinforcing a pattern of increased psychological needs as the families and individuals move away from traditional Costa Rican attitudes and behaviors. These value orientations are both cultural and familial perceptions of satisfactory health behavior, in that family values are informed and changed by cultural values and societal norms.

In order to fully understand health behavior in Costa Rica, one further level of analysis must be included—the examination of medical institutional structure and its impact on doctor-patient interaction. The patient has been presented in the context of the urban health care system, and the family. However, it is the medical consultation which finally determines patient satisfaction. Possibly it is because of the immediacy of the therapeutic relationship or perhaps it is the dependency of Costa Ricans on medical services. Nonetheless, a perceived therapeutic success relies on satisfactory doctor-patient interaction.

CHAPTER IV

MEDICAL INSTITUTIONS AND DOCTOR-PATIENT INTERACTION

There have been many studies of patient satisfaction and medical compliance (Davis 1968, 1971; Korsch et.al. 1968; Ordonez Plaja et.al. 1968; Freeman et al. 1971; Friedson 1973; Larsen and Rootman 1976; Mechanic 1976; Svarstad 1976; Locker and Dunt 1978) all of which demonstrate the importance of doctor-patient interaction and communication as determinants in adequate health care delivery. Kleinman (1978) has expanded this discussion by bringing attention to the importance of individual and cultural explanatory models of clinical processes in determining appropriate health behavior.

Changes in economic and political systems have also been shown to impact the success of health care through inconsistencies in health care structure (Lasker 1977), the development of interest group coalitions (Alford 1975), and inequalities of resource allocations (Janzen 1978). Other studies employ a macroanalysis of power and authority as well as a microanalysis of clinical setting to provide a more inclusive model of health systems and health process (Field 1973; Elling 1978; Janzen 1978; Waitzkin 1979; Frankenberg 1980). Further, studies of political ideology in developing countries suggest that there is a direct relationship between these countries' ideologically based health policies and inadequate health care delivery (Mburu 1981; de Miguel 1977; Pearce 1980). The reliance on physicians' professional values to define national health care needs has created urban, hospital-based medical systems which ignore the overwhelming national problems of sanitation, nutrition, and rural health care (Ugalde 1980, Navarro 1978);

The study of doctor-patient interaction in Costa Rican outpatient clinics explores the relationship of patient dissatisfaction and interactional style by integrating the interactional data with an analysis of institutional and ideological factors. Patient behavior, physician performance, and social interaction in the medical consultation are found to be influenced by the institutional and political setting. A comparison of the differences in medical institutional ideology and in doctor-patient interaction explicates the relationship of medical institutional politics to success of the therapeutic encounter.

The patient perspective was obtained in the second phase of the research project, during which the observed patients were also interviewed before and after the consultation. The questions and examples of responses were presented in the previous chapter.

The Public Health Institution

The Ministry of Public Health—renamed the Ministry of Health in 1973—is an executive governmental agency whose chief administrator is appointed by the President. The Ministry defines national health policy and organizes and coordinates the health services of the country. An extensive preventive medicine program which includes control of the importation and use of drugs and preservation of the environment is maintained in order to protect personal health (Ministerio de Salubridad Publica 1973: 4–5).

Until October 3, 1973 when a law was passed transferring all public hospitals to the Social Security administration, the Ministry also provided free or low-cost medical assistance to persons not protected by the Social Security system or insured by the Instituto Nacional de Seguros, an autonomous government agency that handles workmen's compensation and private insurance cases. To fulfill these various functions the Public Health system in 1973 directed 62 community clinics, 10 mobile clinics that travelled to remote regions, 205 nutrition and education centers, 10 nutrition recuperation centers, 52 dental clinics, 13 rural assistance centers, 27 rural dispensaries, 19 rural health posts and 15 hospitals. Six hundred and thirty-five doctors, 588 nurses, 2,009 aides and other professionals staff these facilities (Ministerio de Salud 1974: 7).

Hospital San Juan de Dios, the oldest and largest Public Health hospital in San José, is governed by a board of trustees appointed by the Junta de Protección Social de San José; the board is composed of distinguished community members who advise the hospital in its social responsibility under the auspices of the

Ministry. For over 40 years, a single physician has served as director of both the administrative and medical treatment sectors and the liaison between the board of trustees and the hospital (1973 interview). The income from national lottery and soccer betting, a portion of the general sales tax, and 4.5% of the national budget allotted to health, finance the rising costs of hospitalization: $14.50 per hospital day and $5.50 per outpatient consultation in 1973 (Ministerio de Salud 1975). An average of $0.12 per hospital day of these costs are paid by the patient. Patients pay according to their ability to do so; the public registry of land and property ownership is investigated and income plus possessions are used to calculate the patient donation. In January 1973, 11% of all patients paid the full cost of treatment, 53% paid a part and 35% paid nothing. Of the 11% who paid, 8% stayed in the private wing, *pension*, of the hospital and paid separate doctor, nursing, room, and board fees. San Juan de Dios serves the entire country in specialties not locally available and is the principle public inpatient and outpatient facility. Inpatient and outpatient service statistics are presented in Table V.

Table V
Hospital Service Comparison for January 1973

	Public Health[1]		*Social Security*[2]	
Inpatient	*San Juan de Dios*	*Chapui*	*Calderon Guardia*	*Mexico*
Number of beds	1024	1037	509	709
Occupancy	90%	92%	72.3%	80.3%
Outpatient				
Average number of consultations	525/day	78/day	996/day	827/day
Total number of doctors	147	11	155	216
Average number of patients seen	6.3/hour	2.5/hour	3.6/hour	3.3/hour

[1] Ministerio de Salud, Deparamento de Estadística 1974.

[2] Caja Costarricense de Seguro Social, Departmento de Actuarial y Estadístico 1974.

Patients enter the hospital in four ways: (1) seriously ill patients go directly to emergency, (2) patients are referred to a specialty clinic by a private doctor, (3) patients are referred by another clinic in the same system because the clinic does not offer the required specialist, or (4) patients self-refer and enter the *consulta extemporanea* outpatient service. Outpatients at San Juan de Dios may wait an entire day, standing in a line to see a doctor, or may be required to return the next day.

The nurses report that they try to see those patients who have travelled the farthest first. The consultation room is very small and noisy as the nurse fights with waiting patients to remain outside the door. Sometimes the patient starts speaking immediately without responding to the doctor's introductory "*Que le paso*?" or "*Que es lo que tiene*?" ("What happened?" or "What do you have?"). The patient speaks rapidly, listing a series of symptoms modified by descriptions of the kind and duration of the pain. The doctor generally nods, writing as he listens, and rarely touches or examines the patient. The doctor may smile or joke in response to some friendly gesture by the patient, but usually the doctor makes his diagnosis, and gives instructions on proper medication and conduct for successful treatment. Most examinations are brief, two to four minutes, and the entire consultation often lasts only a few minutes more.

At Hospital San Juan de Dios the doctor is contracted for a morning or an afternoon to see as many patients as possible, or as many as are waiting. The number of patients seen, therefore, varies with the number waiting or with the number scheduled and was observed to range from four to thirty consultations with an average of 6.3 per hour. The tone of the consultation also depends on the number of patients and the press of those outside, so that a doctor may take more time to give instructions and answer questions when fewer patients are around. Patients may make appointments to see a particular doctor, but most often see the one who is available at the time.

In the Public Health clinics, the nurse and doctor work together to try to see everyone and attend to their problems. Although the doctors appear brusque, their observed actions were usually to speed the patient on his way. There was a personal camaraderie among those working in one area which the patients could see and respond to; patients often tried to use that relationship to encourage the nurse to tell the doctor something on their behalf. The nurse also makes the doctor's appointments in the same office unless the patient was referred and would consult the doctor if there was at any time conflict or patient confusion. Drugs are dispensed at a nearby counter so that patients stay in one area.

The Hospital Psiquiátrico Manuel Antonio Chapui is a Public Health psychiatric facility. About half the inpatients have chronic disorders and live there; some patients have been residents for more than 20 years. Other patients visit the hospital in the mornings for food and medication because the family is too poor to adequately support the patient or because the patient has been abandoned. Chapui, as Costa Rica's only chronic care psychiatric hospital in 1973, is similar in size and occupancy to San Juan de Dios, but has a much smaller outpatient service and provides only specialty patient care (Table V). A new psychiatric facility has been completed recently outside the city and has replaced Chapui's central role in caring for chronic and acute mental illness.

The psychiatric service waiting area is filled with rows of people on benches facing one another, talking and sharing lunches, advising one another on how to take medication or produce a cure, or waiting in line for the pharmacy. A male secretary calls out patients' first names, instructs patients to pick up their charts from "Don Edgar" and then go in to see the doctor. The consultation varies in length and style from a first visit, when the doctor asks a long series of medical history questions and makes his diagnosis, to the brief and familiar interaction of a patient in treatment who has come to renew prescribed medications. Chapui's outpatient service is popularly known for its friendly atmosphere and personal attention that is possible in the limited context of a specialty hospital.

The Social Security Institution

The Costa Rican Fund for Social Security (Caja Costarricense de Seguro Social) in 1973 covered 60.2% of the nation and 50.2% of the workers in the economically active sector. Within the next ten years, by law, Social Security must extend its medical and dental assistance, hospitalization, pharmaceutical services, sick pay, and burial benefits to the entire country with 75% of the population reported as covered by 1980 (Caja Costarricense de Seguro Social, Sección de Relaciones Publicas 1973; Casas and Vargas 1980).

Social Security employee coverage in 1973 was 30% in social and personal services, 20% in industry, 17% in agriculture, 14% in business, 7% in construction, 5% in transportation, 7% other (Caja Costarricense de Seguro Social, Departamento de Actuarial y Estadístico 1974) with the participation rate higher in office or factory-oriented occupations and lower among independent workers. To qualify for Social Security benefits cited above, a worker pays 4% (plus an additional 1% on income in excess of US $360) of the monthly salary, the employer contributes 5%, and the State 2%; if there is no employer the individual must pay both employee and employer shares. The subscriber may also allot an additional 2.5%, the employee another 2.5%, and the State 2% to accrue disability, old age and pension rights for the surviving spouse. The pension amounts to monthly payments of 70% of the first $36 of the pensioner's monthly salary and a diminishing percentage of each additional $36 per month earned (Caja Costarricense de Seguro Social 1971).

A recent report states that Social Security benefits are now available to the uninsured (Harrison 1981) and an anthropological observer recently commented that local residents use the Social Security clinics whether or not they are paying for the benefits (Michael Whiteford, personal communication). Casas and Vargas (1980) and Rosenberg (1981) both discuss the various changes in taxation, quotas and calculation of patient coverage which have occurred many times during the history of the service. I am reporting the requirements which were in practice during the 1972 to 1974 field study and which applied to patients observed in these institutions.

Disability, old age and death insurance was carried by 45.3% of the total population and 37.8% of the economically active population in 1973 (Caja Costarricense de Seguro Social 1974). Medical and pharmaceutical assistance is provided to the insured worker's family, which includes a wife or companion, children under 18 or students under 22 years of age, mother or father if incapacitated or over 65 years of age, illegitimate children if recognized, and a husband who can not work and depends on a wife who is insured (Caja Costarricense de Seguro Social, Sección de Relaciones Publicas 1973). The structure of Social Security and its benefits were adapted from the Chilean program (Bell 1971: 30), and closely resemble the Spanish Instituto Nacional de Previsión developed during 1938–44, approximately the same time frame as the development of the equivalent program in Costa Rica (Press 1973). Rosenberg (1981) notes that President Calderon Guardia, in order to write the Costa Rican legislation, dispatched Padilla Castro to Chile to study their social security system.

Benefits and limitations of services are carefully listed in the Social Security by-laws, nonetheless some Costa Ricans do not fully understand the complex rules:

> An employer sent his agricultural worker to the Social Security clinic to have a twisted wrist looked at and to have the *peon's* 14 year old daughter's cavities filled. Because the clinic was an hour's bus ride and it was often difficult to go, the father also took another child to have his teeth

> checked. Upon arrival at the clinic, the dentist explained that one child must come back another day as only one family member per day is allowed to visit the dentist. The dentist proceeded to extract the daughter's four front teeth and then explained she would have to come to him privately to have the teeth replaced because Social Security benefits for a family member do not include reconstructive dental work. The father was dismayed; he was poor and his daughter could never marry well without front teeth. He had received a balm for his wrist and was told not to work for 3 days; this meant his employer would have to pay him for the days not worked—Social Security pays for work loss only after the 4th day of inactivity due to illness or injury. They returned home commenting that they wondered why they bothered to even go to the clinic. (Fieldnotes 1974)

Hospital Doctor Rafael Angel Calderon Guardia and Hospital Mexico are administered by the Junta Directiva through the medical directorate of Social Security. Each hospital is headed by a physician and has a staff of over 4,000 employees and 750 doctors (interview 1973). The country is divided into two geographical service sectors: Calderon Guardia serves the eastern zone of Limon, Turrialba, Cartago, and the eastern half of San José; Hospital Mexico serves the western zone of Puntarenas, Guanacaste, Alajuela, and the western half of San José. In addition to these two hospitals, Social Security maintains 5 clinics in San José (one is within Calderon Guardia) and 68 clinics in the outlying areas, in some cases sharing the rural Public Health facilities. If these local community services are insufficient, the patient is referred to one of the two main hospitals in San José. The San José hospitals also have specialty services not found in local clinics: Calderon Guardia directs the psychiatric, tuberculosis, and venereal disease sections; and Hospital Mexico administers psychosomatic medicine and neurosurgery. Special services are being expanded, but many need expensive equipment and technical personnel. The hospitals' desire to have their own facilities to enhance prestige has led to the replication of specialized units that are underutilized and costly to maintain. One example is that both hospitals maintain psychiatric clinics which compete for practitioners and patients.

The hospital system is financed 60.5% by salary deductions, 37.2% by the State's contribution, and the remainder from interest and investments (Caja Costarricense de Seguro Social 1972); 72% of this income is used to defray the cost of hospitalization ($23.70 per hospital day in Calderon Guardia, and $27.50 per hospital day in Hospital Mexico) and outpatient consultation ($5.00 per visit in Calderon Guardia and $5.50 per visit in Hospital Mexico) (Caja Costarricense de Seguro Social, Departamento de Actuarial y Estadístico 1974). The size, occupancy, and services provided in both hospitals is comparable, with Hospital Mexico being slightly larger and treating fewer patients because of its specialty emphasis (Table V).

According to the chief of the Social Security outpatient services, every person sees the same general medicine physician each visit; if the patient comes in without an appointment and demands attention, the patient is seen briefly in the *consulta extemporanea* clinic, where the doctor orders medicines or a referral to the appropriate specialty (Interview 1973). The Calderon Guardia clinic consists of a large central waiting room full of chairs and benches turned away from one another; long administration and receptionist counters run the length of one side of the room, and doctors' offices on two sides open onto the waiting room. The long room echoes with the noise: crying children, patients scolding children, nurses and clerks giving instructions to patients, and employees gathering for coffee and conversation. Richardson and Bode describe the Social Security clinic in Puntarenas:

> People, not infrequently as many as a hundred, crowd into waiting rooms and sit patiently—or impatiently—while the staff scurries about processing their records and establishing contact between the people and doctors. (1971: 258)

The patient enters this room, presents a card and an *orden patronal* (a receipt that certifies that the deductions have been paid for the previous month) to the receptionist who verifies the appointment. The patient then goes to the nurse who works in front of the physician's office; she takes the patient's name and orders the chart. The patient is seated and instructed to enter the consultation room following another patient. The patient is expected to be ready to enter the office immediately after the designated person, and is chastised if slow or forgetful. If the patient is more than 15 minutes late, the appointment is automatically cancelled.

The doctor is contracted to see six patients an hour with an average of 3.6 consultations per hour, however, a wide range of consultation lengths actually occurs. The pace is leisurely; the doctor is generally relaxed and there is time to discuss the patient's problem and possible treatment. After the consultation, the patient returns to the administration counter to request another appointment on the doctor's recommendation. The delay for some specialty appointments may be as long as six months. Finally the patient goes to the pharmacy to pick up the prescribed medicine.

Fragmentation and separation of medical and administrative services is a dominant characteristic of Social Security clinic activities—making an appointment, waiting, seeing the doctor, and getting medication—are located in different places, and the facilitating personnel have limited contact and few opportunities to exchange information. Relationships between doctors and secretaries, nurses and patients, and doctors and nurses reflect a lack of communication and a misunderstanding of rules and responsibilities. Secretaries give patients appointments based on their rules of availability without consulting or considering the doctors' treatment schedule. The doctors cannot understand why patients do not appear in the time period suggested for the next visit. Nurses are teased by doctors for gossiping and accused of being paid for doing nothing. Nurses, however, receive the brunt of patient displeasure; they deal with aggressive patients who verbally abuse them during the long pre-consultation wait and criticize them for any lapse in attention or service.

Medical Institution Comparison

The Public Health and Social Security institutions provide parallel services for inpatient and outpatient health care. The Public Health hospitals are larger in terms of the number of beds and provide more inpatient care, while the Social Security hospitals provide more outpatient consultation (Table V). The ratio of patients to doctors in the various outpatient clinics is also very striking (Table V); however, these differences are minimized when the number of beds is added to the number of consultations representing the total doctor workload. The hospital differences presented in Table V reflect the manpower emphasis on inpatient care at Hospital San Juan de Dios and on outpatient care at Hospital Calderon Guardia. The chronic inpatient population at Hospital Chapui is a special case in that there is little physician care available, while Hospital Mexico functions as a secondary care service which provides a better overall ratio of doctors to patients. The real difference in outpatient care is encoded by the number of patients seen per hour, which is almost twice as large in San Juan de Dios as in Calderon Guardia, and certainly influences the quality of care. These differences in service provision, however, are less striking when contrasted with their ideological differences produced by their distinct histories and political affiliations.

The sociopolitical histories of the Public Health and Social Security institutions account in large part for the basic structural and interactional differences in the observed patient and staff behavior. The histories identify the basic value orientation and political goals of the institutions' founders and describe how these values influence the course of institutional development.

It should be recalled that the public health institutions in Costa Rica evolved from charity services initiated by the Catholic Church and that the religious control of public health was later limited. The impetus for government participation in the creation of a public health hospital was an emerging republicanism stimulated by independence from Spain in 1821, and the advent of coffee production on a large scale, roughly from 1830–1890, which precipitated the formation of an upper class and concomitant concentration of wealth. The wealth accumulated during this period went into the social welfare needs and material progress of the nation (Bell 1971). The rapid growth in coffee production concentrated land, once held by a number of small land owners, in the hands of a few families who had the financial backing for the processing and transport of coffee (Seligson 1980). From this new class emerged the "Generation of 1889," which perpetuated a noblesse oblige tradition through legislative means, establishing universal education and instigating national social reform through public health services. The development of an elite, with both economic means and political power, transferred the traditional religious and upper class concerns of charity, personal security, and welfare ideology to their representatives in the National Legislative Assembly (Stone 1974; Bell 1971). This control was maintained until 1935 when the political power of elite descendents was diluted by economic diversification, immigration, and population growth. The new group was no longer able to mandate social welfare projects (Sancho 1935; Stone 1969, 1974).

The social relationships developed during this period were those of interdependence:

> The success of the enterprise (coffee production) was subject to the productivity of the peon, and this to the paternalistic rapport which the planter could maintain with his scanty labor force. If the peon depended on the planter for his salary and home, the planter depended on the peon for good production, which was the basis of both his wealth and prestige within his own class. (Stone 1974: 408)

The resulting *patron-peon* relationship permeated the interactions of the classes in institutions and activities where services and goods intersected, including the doctor-patient encounter in the public health facilities. The public health hospital became an extension of the *patron-peon* relationship in which doctors were members of the upper class and patients were willing to exchange respect, devotion, and agricultural goods for services that only the upper class could offer.

The later evolution during the 1930's and 1940's of the Social Security institution partly represents this tradition of "an elite" committed to the social welfare and well-being of the citizenry (Rosenberg 1981: 296) but, it was implemented through the efforts of Communist forces working in a voting compromise within the Legislative Assembly.

Costa Rican social relationships were also affected by the social and political ideology reflected in President Calderon Guardia's program of social guarantees of the 1940's. According to historian Bell, "basic human relationships were changed and many felt uncomfortable with the changes: a patron could no longer deal arbitrarily with 'his' workers" (1971: 82). A new ideology of social equality and welfare rights permeated the Social Security system, and its institutional problems reflected the new social alignments and relationships.

The historical ideological differences are further maintained by the physicians who tend to work for the system that is consistent with their political position and social values. During this study and before nationalization, upper-class physicians, particularly those of old landowning families, tended to work in San Juan de Dios. Some felt that Costa Rica would return to a free election medical system and refused to work for a system where a secretary tells the physician who will be seen and when. The Social Security tended to attract middle-class physicians who were socially mobile, with less status and fewer family connections. The life history of a young, aspiring physician reveals how employment in the Social Security is used to accrue the professional status and adequate income which allows the family to then patronize upper-class schools, clubs, and privileges:

> The doctor thought that it was not necessary for his wife to work. He thought that by omitting luxuries they could live only on his salary. But, he added, his wife had set her mind on sending the children to St. Francis High School, and so she also works at the Social Security to pay for the children's education. They are paying off the house they built in an upper-class *barrio* and she also helps her parents with money. (Interview 1974)

Physician recruitment also has been influenced by differential wages and institutional commitment. The Public Health physician was traditionally paid very little and only worked a half a day, reserving the remaining hours for a lucrative private practice. The Social Security physicians are hired for a full day and are expected to work full time. Currently, however, Public Health doctors are said to be paid equivalant salaries to Social Security physicians and the majority (nearly 90%) of doctors are now employed by the Social Security, further reducing salary and class differences. The historically derived class ideologies associated with specific medical institutions may be diminished with nationalization, nonetheless, these differences continue to be played out in distinct doctor-patient interactions within the medical consultation.

Doctor-Patient Interaction

The examination of doctor-patient interaction illustrates how the structural and historical construction of the medical institution is enacted in everyday clinic function and participant behavior. By observing differences in patient attitudes and doctor style in the medical consultations, the impact of ideology on the expected pattern of interaction can be described.

Patient attitude and doctor style have been coded according to characteristic types from the observed clinic consultations. The typology for patient attitude was generated from the data which describe a simple dichotomy between the submissive, shy patients and the confident, demanding patients. The two types are illustrated by patient cases drawn from the consultation data.

The doctor style typology was developed from a study by Ordonez Plaja, Cohen and Samora of outpatient clinic physician-patient communication in urban Columbia. This typology describes the four characteristic styles: 1) bureaucratic and task-oriented, 2) insecure and detailed, 3) self-assured and interpretive, and 4) amiable and expressive (1968: 178). These categories referred to the style by which the physician treated the patient. The bureaucratic physician was concerned with the immediate tasks of diagnosis and disposing of the case, and therefore showed limited sensitivity toward patient feelings and problems. The insecure and detailed physician tended to carry out a lengthy interview and offered prolonged explanations in order to establish rapport. The self-assured and interpretive physician had a sense of correctness about the questions asked and offered interpretations about underlying problems. The amiable, person-oriented physician showed an awareness of the feelings of the patient and the social factors that influence behavior, but appeared to have less insight or flexibility as to the appropriate use of this knowledge.

The typology from the Colombian study was used to code the Costa Rican doctor style with the slight modification of adding authoritarian behavior to the bureaucratic category. Based on the consultation data, authoritarian behavior often accompanied the bureaucratic, task-oriented style of a physician. Illustrations of each of these physician types is presented in the doctor style discussion.

Patient Attitude

Public Health patients were observed to be more submissive, shy and withdrawn in their interaction with the doctor. The following three cases from San Juan de Dios characterize this Public Health institution patient attitude:

> A young man complains of a problem with his eyes. He can see, but he has had pain in both eyes for over 2 years. The doctor examines his eyes. The young man is very shy and does not look up. Doctor questions him many times as if he does not understand or believe the patient. Patient is quite nervous and does not seem to focus on the doctor. Doctor gives him a prescription for conjunctivitis and states that he believes that it is just an infection as the man does not have any trouble seeing.

> A man of 28 says he has stomach pain and has been vomiting for the past 2 days. Doctor examines his stomach. Doctor wants exams done of the stomach area and wants him to come back in a day for the results. Doctor keeps repeating that the patient should come back tomorrow as the patient acts as if it is difficult to understand. Patient acts as if he feels very bad and is confused; he has a great deal of difficulty reading and puts his head on his hands. Doctor says he will give him an injection to stop the vomiting and pain. The doctor keeps an eye on the patient as he writes; he tells him, "Roberto go out and get this injection; you will feel better. Do you understand?" As the patient begins to walk out the doctor says: "Wait, I will also order an x-ray."

> A young woman from a small town outside of San José. Doctor asks if married; she answers no. Doctor asks, "Sexual relations?" Woman answers, "Yes". "OK," says the doctor, "Please undress and get on the examining table." She complains of pain in the vaginal canal, existing since September. Doctor does vaginal examination. Much pain is experienced when she has sexual relations. She grimaces during the

> examination but does not say anything. Doctor refers to gynecologist. Tells me in front of patient that they must investigate for cancer.

In each case, the patient dutifully answers questions and responds minimally to doctor's exam or interaction. The submissive, shy and withdrawn manner of the San Juan de Dios patient is encouraged, if not conditioned, by the doctor. The patient normally passes through only one gatekeeper before reaching the physician. It is the physician, in the medical institutional setting, who maintains the traditional role expectations of the *patron-péon* relationship, and the patient who reinforces this socially acceptable pattern.

In contrast to the Public Health patients, the Social Security patients were observed to be more frequently confident, difficult, and demanding in their interaction with the doctor. The following cases from Hospital Mexico and Calderon Guardia illustrate this difference in patient attitude, when compared to the previous Public Health cases:

> A young woman is seven months pregnant. She starts out by asking the doctor if there is anything that she can give her children so they will not wet the bed at night. The doctor says, "Yes," but she must bring them in to be studied to see what the problem is. The doctor asks her if she is in the prenatal clinic, and he asks how her husband is. She changes the subject. She wants to know if they can perform a vasectomy on her husband. The doctor tells her that they must bring a signed statement of consent for the operation and their reasons for wanting it. She asks about the hospital for having her baby, continually repeating questions. She complains that she did not get to see the baby for two days and she does not want that to happen again. The doctor assures her that it will not. She asks how long she will be in the hospital. She will be there for three days with natural child birth and two more if she has anesthesia, the doctor answers her.

> The patient is not much better. He saw another doctor who gave him pills. He was riding a motorcycle but can no longer continue because he loses his balance. He must now ride the bus to his job in the electric company. The patient asks for a permanent work leave, but the doctor says he will give him only three months. The patient then adds that yesterday he fell in the bathtub. The doctor examines him by having him shut his eyes, turn around and the open his eyes. He does not fall. The patient complains that the pills do not work; the doctor reduces the dosage because the pills make the patient more dizzy. The patient also requests a dandruff prescription, but the doctor tells him to come back in three months for a check-up. He also orders exams.

> The patient inquires about his diabetic curve; the doctor tells him a number of the curve points. The patient then asks if he should be careful.
>
> An older woman with a very bad cough. Saturday she went to the emergency room for help. They gave her an injection. In a condemning voice she says that the doctor had given her medication, but that it did not work. She has had two attacks since her last appointment. Doctor asks her how long has she had asthma? Patient replies, "for a little time."

The demanding attitude of the Social Security patient is characteristic of patients in pre-paid group practices. Freidson reports three kinds of demanding patients: those with complaints for which there is little the physician can do or for which he can find no cause, those who attempt to use "pull" to obtain services, and those who demand services as a contractual right. The kind of demanding patient most often found in the Social Security clinics is identified as the most difficult for the physician to deal with because: "they posed demands which the physicians were unaccustomed to dealing with, for the demands stemmed from the contractual framework of practice" (1973: 484–483).

The difference in patient attitude may indeed be attributed to the mode of payment. One Social Security physician comments that:

> They come in for every symptom, because they pay they feel that they must get their money out of the system and do not understand that the payments are to cover major medical expenses when needed. In San Juan de Dios they are more patient and less demanding because they know they are not paying. (Interview 1973)

Goffman, in his analogy of doctoring as a tinkering service, suggests that when the doctor (the server) performs major services for very poor clients, the server may feel that charging no fee is more dignified than a reduced fee. The server thus avoids dancing to the clients' tune, or even bargaining, and is able to show that he is motivated by a disinterested involvement in his work (1961: 327). Extending this analogy, then, the prepaid patient would have the right to demand attention as the server has been paid a fixed sum for unlimited service. The prepayment aspect of the Social Security clinic provides one explanation for the confident, demanding attitude of patients. However, doctor style and patient role expectations based on the ideological social equality of the participants influence the course of doctor-patient interaction in a different and more direct manner.

Doctor Style

Doctor style tends to be the most sensitive indicator of medical institution sociopolitical structure. Doctor style was significantly more bureaucratic and authoritarian in the Public Health clinics (Table VI). A consultation interaction was directed, oriented towards making a diagnosis and referring the patient:

> A grey haired woman of about 56. She has a pain in her chest, back, and waist. Has had the flu (*grippe*) for 15 days. The pain is strong in her head and eyes. Doctor states that she has *grippe* complicated by sinusitis. She went to the doctor in Alajuela, but he sent her here without an order; he just told her to go. Doctor asks why she did not use the local Public Health clinic (*unidad sanitario*). She answers it is only open every 15 days. Doctor asks for other symptoms. She says that she has a cough with yellow phlegm. Her throat also seems to close on her when she talks. Doctor takes her temperature, listens to her chest, ordering her to "take that thing off," to get the patient to take off her blouse. Doctor gives her medicine and a referral appointment.

Table VI
Doctor Style of Interaction by Medical Institution

Doctor Style	*Public Health*		*Social Security*		*Total Sample*	
	N	%	*N*	%	*N*	%
Bureaucratic, Authoritarian	90	53.9	76	34.9	166	43.1
Self-assured, Interpretative	53	31.7	88	40.4	141	36.6
Amiable, Expressive	21	12.6	43	19.7	64	16.6
Insecure, Detailed	3	1.8	11	5.0	14	3.6
Total	167	100.0	218	100.0	385[1]	100.0

$X^2 = 15.519$ d.f. = 3 SIG. = 0.001

[1] This number does not respresent the entire 457 observed consultations as a number of consultations had to be dropped from the sample because they did not respresent a completed doctor-patient interaction. These cases included patients who came by to ask advice, but who were not seen; patients who came in to have forms signed or filled out; patients who came in for school exams, and other cases where the data was not comparable to the illness presentation/treatment model of the majority of interactions.

In the Social Security clinics, doctor style tends to be more self-assured, interpretative, and amiable (Table VI). The doctors appear interested in engaging the patient in conversation, eliciting social details, and offering interpretation of both the patient's medical and social problems. A consultation from Calderon Guardia illustrates the self-assured, interpretive doctor style:

> A woman of 52. Patient says, "I am well and without medicine." Came in to know about an exam for blood sugar; the doctor says that her exam is good. She asks about the *grippe* that she had had. She says that she is in treatment for high blood pressure and now also has hot flashes (*calores*). Doctor examines her blood pressure and says that she is much better. Doctor asks if her high blood pressure is associated with a family problem. She answers that yes, her husband was quite sick and had an operation here in the Social Security hospital. He is better now. He is still losing weight however.

Doctor style in the Social Security clinic may also be amiable but less successful in terms of understanding the underlying factors in the patient illness:

> Young man from Turrialba who now lives in San José. Doctor says to him "you are well are you not?" and repeats when finally the patient answers "No, I am not. I still have the same problem of the gastritis; there was a time when it was better." He has an intestinal inflammation, the patient says. Doctor explains to him that the problems make it worse, but the patient goes on that he has had it so long. Doctor responds that he had said that it was better, and the patient reacts again, "Yes, but still it is bad." He has had a *novia* (girlfriend) but is not thinking of marriage. Sees his family. Has gas and burning pain, does not vomit but feels as if he is going to. Lemon and milk hurt him to drink. "And the injections?" asks the doctor. "The injections were good," he says. Doctor examines the patient as he complains of pain. Patient asks if the doctor can not give him the injections; that he is tired of all the pills. Doctor gives him injections and a diet. Again the doctor asks if the patient has noticed getting better and patient says that he still complains of sinus irritation. Doctor orders x-ray of the nasal passage. Patient says it hurts with sun. Doctor gives him drops for his nose.

The analysis of the historical development of the medical institutions suggests that the Public Health doctors employ a bureaucratic approach with patients in response to the charity orientation of the hospital and the tradition of the upper-class doctor bestowing services without charge on the poor patient. The hierarchical doctor-patient roles are reinforced by the hospital orientation, physician recruitment, and the class differentiation of the patients. An authoritarian style develops in this situation where the socioeconomic and intellectual superiority of the doctor can be overtly manipulated:

> Man, 45, from Guancaste. He speaks very low. He has a pain in his stomach. For the last 8 days has not been well. At first, he reports that the color of his stools had changed from black to purple. Doctor continues to question in curt tone. Doctor asks how the man knows what color his stools are if he eliminates in a hole. The patient, very embarrassed, says that sometimes he eliminates in the fields and therefore notices, but says that the color did not change and that the stools were still the same color. The patient has never been in the hospital. Doctor roughly examines the patient, and continues to ask, "What kind of work do you do?" "Do you drink the water where you live?"

The physicians who work in the Public Health clinics also reinforce a charity doctrine in their feelings about patients:

> They (San Juan de Dios patients) appreciate what you are doing for them. The poor people bring me eggs and chickens because I am not ashamed to carry home a *bolsa* (shopping bag). They are so grateful. (Interview 1974)

In the Social Security clinics the ideology of social equality is reflected in an interpretaive and amiable doctor style. Nonetheless, doctor discomfort indicates that there are problems involved in the adjustment to social equality in the physician role. Some doctors respond in a detailed and insecure style in which the doctor is overly solicitous, investigates every comment and symptom, and hesitates to give either advice or diagnosis. Doctor interviews corroborate the observation conclusions; dissatisfaction, frustration, and anger at the Social Security system, and complaints centering on the difficult, demanding patients, and their inability to control their hours, appointments or patients, characterize their discussions. A summary of a coffee break discussion during an afternoon of consultation reports that:

> Doctors are frustrated as there is not time for treatment of the patient. Doctors are bored with their work. Their satisfaction comes from their private practice. Maybe it is because before doctors all had public consultations as well as upper-class patients; then the Social Security began. Doctors felt that the Social Security would not succeed, but it is growing in size and coverage. A majority of doctors work for the institution, but they do not have the same relations with their patients. Patients in Social Security do not know how to use the system. When they demand services which

> the doctor does not like, the doctor rejects the patient even more. The system does not work, but of course it is the patient who suffers. Both the patient and the doctor are unhappy and the system will continue to cover everyone in the country without satisfying anyone. The question is how to change the system so that it can work for the participants. (Fieldnotes 1973)

A doctor who has worked in both systems comments:

> The patient of the Caja comes to use the clinic when he does not have anything, but the error is compounded when the doctor does not examine the patient and tells him that he has nothing, just giving him a prescription. The doctor is telling the patient who feels some discomfort that he does not, which only makes the situation worse. It would be better if the doctor would examine the patient and tell him that he does not find anything physical, but that the problem could be related to some problem in his life. This approach would reduce the misunderstanding.
>
> The traditional view of San Juan de Dios came from private practice. The doctors were paid very little to give their time, and now they are paid the same as doctors in Social Security and want to have salaries. Many doctors hold 2-3 jobs within the same time period which means the patient does not receive the doctor's full attention.
>
> The problem between the insured person and the doctors is that the insured have rights but don't have obligations. Politics also influences what happens so that the president goes to open a new clinic and tells people that this is yours and you must make it work, but does not say what their responsibility is to the Social Security clinic. The patient enters the clinic and first encounters the administrator, then the nurse, and the receptionist and fights with each of them. Finally, when the patient arrives at the doctor, he is furious. (Interview 1973)

The two basic patterns of doctor-patient interaction correspond to the two medical institutions. In the Social Security clinics the consultation is characterized by a difficult and demanding patient and an interpretive and amiable physician. The Public Health clinic consultation is one of a bureaucratic, authoritarian physician and a submissive, shy patient. These contrasting modes of interaction are best explained by the sociopolitical context of the individual institutions, further influenced by the mode of payment and organizational setting of the hospital clinics. Interactional patterns are further reinforced by the differences in doctors' workload in the outpatient clinics. These different interactional processes can be evaluated by comparing patient compliance and satisfaction in the two institutions.

Patient Satisfaction

In consultation, interview, and conversation, Social Security patients complain that the wait for services is extremely long, the medicine is not good, and the doctors are inattentive. Compared to Public Health patients who have fewer complaints, the Social Security patients expressed displeasure during the consultation: seven patients directly criticized doctors, nine commented on the long wait, and fifteen said that the medication prescribed was worthless. Some of the complaints by Social Security patients are certainly valid; there should be changes in the scheduling of appointments and the comfort of the waiting area. When comparing research observations by institution, however, these complaints do not differentiate clinic function. The wait is long in all clinics. The doctors in the Public Health hospitals have even less time to give attention to patients and do so in a brusque manner. The same medicines are used by both institutions, and both pharmacies dispense drugs in unmarked metal and plastic containers or brown glass bottles which are relatively inexpensive and encourage the doctor to give dosage instructions. The comparative cost of medicine is also nominal, though slightly higher in the Social Security if calculated as part of the total deduction. Yet the complaints concerning medication are directed at the Social Security and not the Public Health facilities.

The complaints about the Social Security medicine may well be a response to a consultation interaction perceived as difficult and frustrating. The Social Security patients are in a relationship with a doctor who is supposed to consider the patient his or her social equal, treat the patient with respect, and satisfy the patient's demands. Both the patient and the doctor, though, are aware of the sociocultural reality that they almost always occupy different social and economic statuses; the few upper-class patients use private practitioners or travel to the United States for treatment. The consultation, then, becomes a conflicted interaction of compromise and negotiation of the social reality. The actual situation and the expectations of social equality complicate the physician's ability to fulfill his or her culturally prescribed doctoring role and alienate the patient by the absence of expected behavior and role performance. The patient does not directly attack the doctor because of dependence on the medical services, but instead vents dissatisfaction and alienation indirectly through blaming a prescribed medication as ineffective. Mechanic suggests that even in the United States:

> Patients tend to have ambivalent attitudes about physicians. They feel extremely dependent on physicians when they anticipate or have serious illness; they also feel some resentment about their dependence and the authority of the physician. This is perhaps exemplified by the tendency to speak favorably about one's personal physician, but to be critical of physicians in general. Underlying this ambivalence are often very high and somewhat unrealistic expectations of the physician and excessive criticism of any failures to live up to this ideal image. (1976: 172)

In the Costa Rican Social Security clinic, patients' expectations are further complicated by the conflicting social ideology and social reality of the institution. Camacho and Alfaro (1977) discuss the so called "dehumanization of medical attention" and its relation to the Social Security through an historical analysis of Costa Rican social relations, further illustrating the apparent contradictions of a system which provides excellent health care, but which also maintains aspects of social inequality inherent in the clinical situation.

Another explanation for the breakdown in patient satisfaction is offered by Kleinman in his analysis of "institutionalized conflicts between lay and practitioner views of clinical reality and therapeutic success" (1978: 87). The process by which differences in the explanatory models of patient and practitioner create obstacles to effective health care is referred to as "cultural iatrogenesis" (1978: 87). In terms of the Costa Rican example, cultural iatrogenesis is occurring with departure from traditional doctor-patient roles to an ideological system that reorients the social status relationships within the consultation. Further, Larsen and Rootman (1976) suggest that satisfaction with medical care is influenced by the degree to which physician performance corresponds to patient expectations. If patients expect doctors to behave in a traditional doctor role, the interpretative style may in fact negatively influence patient satisfaction.

Richardson and Bode discuss the differences of explanatory models of clinical reality in terms of the relative social position of the healer and patient. The curer and patient are of the same social rank facilitating communication through the similar clinical expectations and creating a symmetrical therapeutic relationship. However,

> the relationship between the physician and patient is asymmetrical. Carmen (an informant) addresses the physician with the formal *usted* ; he replies with intimate *vos*. . . . The physician asserts his authority over the curing process and claims that through his superior knowledge he can cure the ills that cause the patient pain. (1971: 270–71)

The undermining of the physician's authority without changing the mode of communication may in fact reduce the possibility of a successful therapeutic encounter.

Other factors that mediate a successful treatment relate to the amount and kind of information the patient receives about the type of treatment to be administered (Svarstad 1976). The failure of the physician to give adequate information concerning medication and treatment reduces patient adherence to the prescribed treatment regime. Inadequate information about treatment in the Social Security clinic, then, enhances the patient's dissatisfaction expressed in a reluctance to accept prescribed medication. While Costa Rican patient dissatisfaction can primarily be attributed to institutional ideological differences, other factors related to communication and setting must be included in a final explanation.

The Social Security and Public Health institutions no longer exist in the form studied. The 1973 health laws transferred all medical assistance responsibilities to Social Security and recreated a Ministry of Health (the former Ministry of Public Health) which would coordinate health services and focus on developing a preventive health program. As the Social Security institution takes over the Public Health clinics, the structural influences on consultation will change. In light of the research presented here, patient dissatisfaction and problems with patient compliance may increase with the transfer of administrative authority and medical responsibilities from the Public Health to the Social Security system.

CHAPTER V

HEALTH POLICY IMPLICATIONS

The medical anthropological study of Costa Rica began with the intention of demonstrating the importance of cultural and family values in determining health behavior. The anthropological literature of Latin America convincingly argued that family, as the basic culture-bearing unit, was the decisive element in choosing health care strategies and in directing health care change.

The research did confirm the centrality of culture and family in the study of health behavior, however, the unexpected conclusion is that the institutional and political setting is equally powerful. Medical institutions and professional medical roles are often considered as the context in which cultural values are enacted, rather than viewed as part of a sociopolitical process that interacts with health culture norms to produce health behavior. Thus, institutional and ideological criteria, as well as family and cultural factors, must be included in the design of any health care project. Inclusion of an institutional level of analysis in the traditional concerns of medical anthropology has become necessary.

Health and health care are primary cultural concerns in Costa Rica. Costa Ricans engage in complex health seeking behavior, exploiting the folk, popular, and professional health sectors for diverse health services. As the nation has developed from a republic, dominated by families of a ruling elite, to a democratic, representative government, the major medical systems have changed from charity to Social Security institutions offering more Costa Ricans hospital based and preventive health care. Economic growth and technological advances have stimulated investment in the health sector as part of social reform programs. The process of development has medicalized Costa Rican health culture such that the expanded medical care sector now encompasses most functions of a social welfare system.

Under the impact of rapid technological and social change in the urban center of Costa Rica, San José, some institutional structures have expanded in response to social demand, while others have contracted or reformed to accommodate new functions and relationships. These changes are reflected in changing patterns of social interaction and social structure which are described by the study of medical institutions and the urban health system.

Health Care Delivery in Developing Nations

Health care and the delivery of medical services in developing nations are burdened with problems of rapid population growth, malnutrition, poor sanitation systems, and an unequal distribution of medical services (Fendall 1972). Some developing countries suffer from a shortage of medical and environmental resources, while others have adequate manpower and supplies at the national level, but these resources are available only in urban centers, inaccessible to the comparably larger, underserved rural population (Ugalde 1980). The urban-centered health care systems are often staffed by professionals trained in industrialized countries with technological solutions and medical theories which are inappropriate, and in many cases, not economically feasible, for the treatment of indigenous populations. Patients who receive treatment often find it unsatisfying, not fulfilling local expectations and needs (Maclean 1966).

Latin American developing countries partially represent this general description of inadequate resources and services. However, in a number of ways the medical care situation and its problems are distinct. An analysis of international trends in medical care organization places Latin America with European countries having strong medical professions and social security schemes. The independence of systems and lack of coordination of services characterize health care delivery in these countries (Bridgman 1972). The separation of medical and indigenous or paramedical services is reinforced by the bureaucratization of medical services into national health care systems (Press 1973).

The case of Central American nations is somewhere between the Latin American and the prototypical developing country models. Central American countries range from highly pluralistic societies with culturally important indigenous, European, and Caribbean populations, such as Guatemala, to relatively homogenous, European dominated cultures, such as Costa Rica. The problems in health care, thus, vary from the need to integrate indigenous and Western healing traditions (Cosminsky and Schimshaw 1980) [also reported for African countries (Asuni 1979; Good et al. 1979; Green 1980)] to the desire to reduce physician control and the domination of health policy by professional medicine values (Ugalde 1980).

Health care policy in the developing country of Costa Rica emphasizes issues of professional medicine's control of resources, (Friedson 1970; Navarro 1978) and the impact of medical domination at the level of doctor-patient interaction (Waitzkin 1979; Frankenberg 1980). The Costa Rican patient perspective, however, focuses on the importance of the use of multiple therapies and the maintenance of a pluralistic medical system (Nichter 1980). The combination of Costa Rican medical system and patient analyses covers the spectrum of problems experienced in most developing nations.

Research studies of the organization of medical care and health care reform identify political and economic changes as having the major effect on health care structure (Pearce 1980; Unschuld 1979). Health policy in developing nations is sensitive to current political ideologies (Mburu 1981); these ideologies generate health reform models and determine their health care implementation plans (de Miguel 1977). The clearest ideological conflicts develop in colonial situations where there are differences in the perception of health sector needs of the indigenous population and the colonial power (Lasker 1977), and in the historical context of the evolution of medical systems (Field 1980). Medicine responds to current ideologies and the goals of society and thus beomes an indicator of cultural and societal change (Englehardt 1976; Pellegrino 1963).

The study of Costa Rican medicine, culture, and politics contributes to an understanding of the health care problems of developing nations through an examination of the interrelation of health care structure, patient perspective of therapies, and the history of ideological and cultural change. The problems of developing nations are complex, in the sense that there are many levels of dysfunction and discontinuity among the cultural expectations of the individual, the evolving social institutions and the political development of the national government. A multilevel approach to the study of health behavior in these settings, therefore, most accurately approximates the actual structure and process of the health care system.

Anthropological methods provide an opportunity for a study of health care delivery that integrates individual process and institutional structure. The focus is the patient in the role of actor within the medical system. As the patient defines the illness, decides upon a course of action, submits to treatment, and evaluates the results, a health-seeking process within a health care system is described. The description of actor and system creates a model of health behavior upon which health policy recommendations can be made that are appropriate to patients and the medical institutions.

A Model of Health Behavior

The study of Costa Rican health behavior combines analyses of health-seeking strategies, family context, and doctor-patient interaction with the broader concerns of the evolution of medical systems in developing countries and their impact on the therapeutic process. This integration of behavioral and sociocultural levels is characteristic of medical anthropological models of explanation.

Medical anthropology, since its inception, has studied health care as part of an ethnographic context. Health care systems are cultural systems (Kleinman 1978): the rules of analysis are the same as those employed in more general ethnography. The concept of health culture in medical anthropology is employed to describe the ethnographic content of health behavior. Weidman (1979) defines health culture as all the phenomena related to the maintenance of well-being and problems of sickness with which people cope in traditional ways within their own social networks. She includes both the cognitive and social systems, belief and practice, in the health culture domain. Health culture descriptions provide a framework of rules and meanings for culturally appropriate health behavior.

Many models of health behavior, however, do not focus on the cultural definitions of health; instead they emphasize the sick role and social aspects of illness behavior and medical care. (Parsons 1958; Kasl and Cobb 1966; Foster 1978; Segall 1976; Idler 1979). The variations in health behavior are explained by differences in educational level (Croog 1961), medical orientation (Suchman 1964; Farge 1978), religion (Mechanic 1963), self-concept (Kassebaum and Baumann 1965), sexual status (Nathanson 1977; Verbrugge 1978), social class (Hollingshead and Redlich 1958), and referral network (Zola 1973). These studies are predominantly sociological, based on research within the

United States. Cultural concerns are included in these models as differences in illness behavior were observed between ethnic groups (Zborowski 1952; Mechanic 1966; Zola 1966; Wolff and Langley 1968) and in relation to cultural role expectations (Townsend and Carbone 1980).

Medical anthropological contributions to health behavior models have expanded the sociological and psychosocial variables and introduced the concepts of dual use (Press 1969) and hierarchy of resort in curative practices (Romanucci Schwartz 1969). Studies of health behavior outside of the United States have consistently reported the use of many health care strategies in any one illness episode. Dual use (Press 1969; Garrison 1977), the concurrent use of a physician and a curer for treatment of an illness, and hierarchy of resort, the order in which a patient chooses such treatment (Romanucci Schwartz 1969; Colson 1971; Nichter 1978) are constructs generated by the anthropologist to account for cross-cultural aspects of health behavior. Cultural patterns of health care utilization stimulated further research on why indigenous practitioners heal successfully (Kleinman and Sung 1979) and how indigenous healing practices benefit the patient (Finkler 1980; Heggenhougen 1980; Ness 1980). These perspectives are integrated in studies of changing medical situations, in which alternative curing strategies are examined through evaluations of medical resource availability (Woods 1977), and explained by generating models of natural decision making (Debacher 1979; Young 1980, 1981).

Studies of doctor-patient interaction and patient satisfaction also have added to an understanding of health behavior. Research indicates that the fulfillment of social needs (Kurella 1979), the physician assignment procedure (Gray 1980), the personal characteristics of the physician (Locker and Dunt 1978; Woolley et al. 1978), and the degree to which physician performance corresponds to patient expectations (Larsen and Rootman 1976) influence the patient's reported satisfaction with medical care. The variability of patient response and the fact that 80% of patients interviewed report satisfaction (Lebow 1974) suggest the difficulty of interpreting these results without specific contextual data.

The health seeking process as described by Noel Chrisman integrates the social and cultural factors that influence health behavior. In his model cultural factors influence patient symptom definition at the beginning of the illness episode, while social factors predominate during referral and treatment action. Finally, the degree of sociocultural integration determines patient adherence to the prescribed regimen (1977:358). He concludes that:

> The quality of doctor-patient transactions and the degree of adherence, is enhanced by specific practitioner attention to explanatory models, role constraints, and the views and influence of lay consultants. (1977:371).

His model adds the new dimension of explaining patient behavior in terms of the entire illness episode, and in predicting adherence based on the influence of the successful integration of social and cultural factors.

The research on Costa Rican health behavior places this health seeking process in the broader perspective of the institutional, ideological, and political framework of medical care. The proposed multilevel model of health behavior describes the influence of each level on patient behavior through an analysis of patient satisfaction. Patient dissatisfaction is employed as an indicator of therapeutic failure, while reported satisfaction reflects therapeutic success. Contextual data clarify and elaborate the patient response, while ethnographic descriptions are used to corroborate the patient interviews. The proposed model by this process is graphically represented in Figure III.

FIGURE III
Costa Rican
Model of Health Behavior

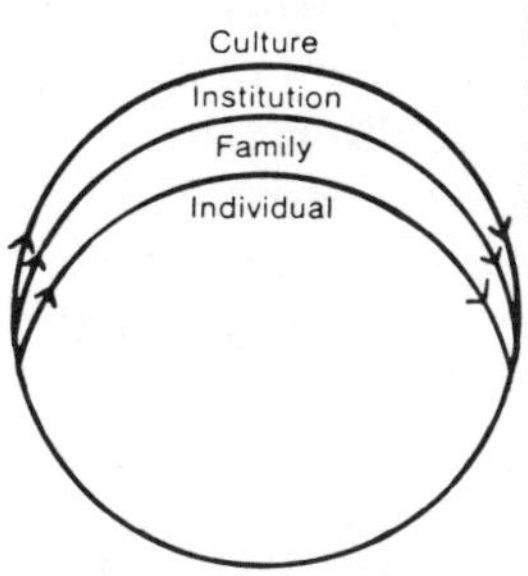

Level	Expression	Process
Culture	Health Culture	Medicalization
Institution	Medical Institution	Political Ideology
Family	Health Sector Utilization	Explanatory Models
Individual	Hierarchy of Resort	Social Organization of Health Care

The model of health behavior is composed of four levels: the individual, familial, institutional, and cultural. These levels are described as influencing health behavior to varying degrees through social processes that order and change the expression of the health care system at the particular level. In other words, the cultural influence on health behavior is expressed through health culture as that system is changed by the process of medicalization. Similarly, the institutional influence is produced by the impact of political ideology expressed in medical institutional structure. The family level influences health behavior by explanatory models of health sector utilization, and the individual influences his own health behaviors through the selection of a hierarchy of resort based on the local social organization of health care. These levels interact with one another and create a series of patterns of health behavior that may apply in different health care situations.

The model of health behavior offers an organization for arranging health care data in a meaningful way. However, the model only becomes explicit with the application of specific research findings. The medical anthropological study of Costa Rica produced detailed data and analyses on each of these health behavior levels. By examining the conclusions of these research findings through the levels of health behavior model, the choices that a patient has in seeking health remediation emerge, producing a more comprehensive description of the Costa Rican health behavior repertoire.

A sequence of health care strategies is utilized by the individual confronted with an illness. The individual first tries home remedies and then the local pharmacy; if these sources are inadequate the person turns to the medical institution and the doctor. The urban health care system is made up of three health sectors: professional, popular, and folk medicine. Utilization patterns cut across these sectors. The individual patient participates in a plural system, making decisions and health care choices which are the basis of the organization of Costa Rican health care. The multiple use of health sectors by individuals is characteristic of plural medical systems; a health-seeking pattern of the individual patient manipulating health care sectors within a specific hierarchy of resort, in an an effort to obtain satisfactory treatment, describes health behavior in a multiple sector health care system.

The family context influences patient explanatory models of the illness episode and appropriate health care behavior. Patient expectations, explanations, and health care utilization reflect these models and therefore predict the therapeutic outcome. Patient satisfaction is achieved when expectations are fulfilled by the physician; non-psychological explanation of etiology and use of all three health sectors further enhance therapeutic success.

Patient satisfaction, however, is not solely determined by family and personal factors. The impact of the institution on doctor style and patient attitude indicates that the sociopolitical history and structure of the institution determine the success of doctor-patient interaction during outpatient consultation. Patient dissatisfaction with the Social Security system is based on expectations of traditional role performance and interactional style which conflict with the social ideology of the institution.

The analysis of the familial, medical institutional, and cultural determinants of health behavior produces an explanation of patient satisfaction which integrates the micro and macro processes of the health care system. At the cultural level, all Costa Ricans value health, have ideas about how it is to be attained and a repertoire of behavioral modes for obtaining treatment. Cultural conformity is reflected in the consistency of health beliefs and behaviors. In the family context, explanatory cognitive models influence health care choices, patient expectation, and explanation, differentiating the generalized, cultural pattern into individuated, family medical orientations. The cultural, familial, and cognitive formation of patient behavior interacts with the sociopolitical development of the medical system at the point where the patient enters the medical institution. Once within the institution, system ideology influences role performance determining therapeutic success. Patient satisfaction begins with a generalized desire for health and a health-seeking repertoire, and is influenced by family expectations which are fulfilled or ignored in a medical institution where both doctor and patient behavior is ultimately determined by the structure of the medical system. Figure IV presents in diagrammatical form the process of the reduction of health behavior repertoire and increasing institutional control of patient health behavior. Individual health behavior has greatest variability when expressed within the broad range of cultural health elements. That behavior is channelled by family selection and segregation of cultural health elements. Family explanatory models are formed; patient expectations and behaviors conform to family patterns. Finally, the patient enters the medical institutional structure where there is still further reduction of behavior modes from the constraints of medical system structure.

Policy Implications for Health Care Delivery

The analysis suggests a number of policy recommendations for the Costa Rican health care delivery. The health care problems in Costa Rica are not derived from the conflict of biomed-

FIGURE IV

The Reduction of Health Behavior Repertoire

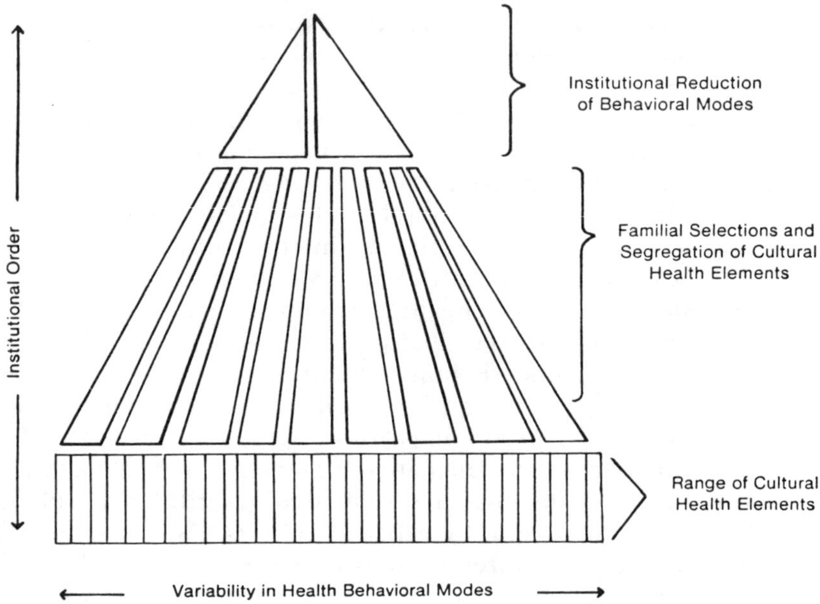

ical and folk models of disease which impedes health care in most cultures. The cultural homogeneity of the country reduces communication problems from the cultural plurality prevalent in larger, more culturally diverse nations. Doctor-patient misunderstanding in Costa Rica is based on acquisition of professional knowledge rather than on cultural differences. Doctors understand folk concepts of illness even though they do not necessarily employ them in consultation with the patient. Health education, then, need not emphasize cultural barriers to communication, but should encourage the already existing pattern.

The plural medical system in Costa Rica provides patients with a variety of health care services and multiple solutions to their health needs. This system works for the patient in the sense that the patient has alternative strategies for each illness episode, that correspond to different explanatory models of causation and treatment. Patients who utilize multiple health sectors are more satisfied with the medical consultation in that the intervention can be more limited since the doctor does not have to respond to all patient needs. Patient demands and expectations therefore more closely correspond to services that the physician can provide. Patient needs not met during the clinic consultation are satisfied in other health settings. In terms of health policy, Costa Rica has legislated that practicing curers, homeopaths, and spiritualists are illegal. Based on data presented, recommendations should be made that these nonprofessional practitioners do provide services valued by patients and that a plural medical system has therapeutic advantages.

The diagram of the reduction of health behavior repertoire (Figure IV) can be employed to indicate appropriate health care intervention strategies and entry points. Consumer satisfaction will increase and quality of care will improve if medical system obstacles that limit health care choice are realigned and the strengths of the system, its cultural hemogeneity and plurality of health services, are reinforced.

The major recommendation from this research focuses on the medical institution and its impact on doctor-patient interaction and therapeutic outcome. It has been observed that interactions in the Social Security clinics are often impeded by role confusion on the part of doctors and patients. Both doctor style and patient attitude do not conform to expectations of role performance. Further, the Social Security system is now nationalized, and the administration is taking over all former Public Health clinics and hospitals. Some adjustment in expectations and translation of ideology into acceptable interaction patterns is necessary in order for patient dissatisfaction not to increase. This will be difficult because the poor quality of interaction is in some sense dependent on the process of social change. As the Costa Rican urban middle class increases, the historical bifurcation of social relations will be minimized. As a transitional solution, workshops and discussions among doctors, patients, and other health clinic staff might lower frustration and interactional tension.

There are also organizational changes that could be made which would enhance Social Security consultation success. As the clinic now functions, services are fragmented when viewed from the patient's perspective. The doctor only orders a treatment, a separate agency distributes the medicine, and another selects a future appointment or referral. If the physician could control return appointments and medicine distribution or at least if the patient could see the linkages among the parts of this therapeutic system, then the physician role as well as patient confidence would be reinforced. Physicians would certainly welcome greater treatment control; although this study has not focused on physician satisfaction, there is interview evidence presented that suggests that physician dissatisfaction affects patient reception. The physicians' ability to fulfill patient expectations would be possible with greater control, thus ultimately increasing patient satisfaction.

The Social Security clinic procedure could be altered to achieve better scheduling or more efficient utilization of physicians' time. This would reduce the amount of waiting time for patients. The present pattern of long coffee breaks in the morning often leaves morning appointments to be taken care of in the afternoon. The long consultations provided by the service do not seem to counteract the frustration built up during the long wait. Other solutions include modifying the number of patients seen, and, an even better remedy, making the waiting time pleasant and constructive. Waiting rooms could provide space for children's play and offer preventive health information or general public health services. These changes aimed at the institutional level of health care services could influence the attitude and expectation of the patient before entering the physician's office.

Recommendations may also be offered at the micro, interactional level of physician consultation. Satisfaction is primarily determined by congruency of expectations. Expectations may be changed externally by education, medical orientation, or socioeconomic access to health resources. Expectations, however, may also be aligned within the consultation by the nature of doctor and patient discussion. If the content of the consultation could emphasize the clarification and negotiation of expectations, doctor-patient communication would be enhanced. In such an exchange, expectations could be openly met or rejected and an explanation offered when treatment is refused. Interpersonal relations rather than institutional structure is the target of this recommendation to improve health care delivery.

The research results of this study suggest that there are certain risks to be considered in the development of nationalized health care systems. These risks may be outweighed by an increase in economic efficiency or access to care in developing countries where medical services are at a premium. Nonetheless, it is important to review the implications of medical system consolidation from the perspective of the Costa Rican data.

The experience in Costa Rica is that the Social Security system will be responsible for all health care services by 1984. This research has explored some of the problems that system has had in providing patients with satisfactory care. The expansion of the Social Security system may exacerbate the problems of highly bureaucratized service and confused doctor-patient interaction. The nationalization of this system may generalize these problems throughout the country. The consolidation of a diversity of systems into one may exaggerate any deficiencies of the original system. Therefore, nationalizing a system without first evaluating that system's weaknesses and deficiencies may create more serious problems when enacted at the national level.

A nationalized health care system also may limit the diversity of care which may be necessary for a medically pluralistic population. The Costa Rican research suggests that patients who use a variety of health care solutions tend to be the most satisfied with the therapeutic outcome. Even in the culturally homogeneous situation of Costa Rica, patients have diverse psychological and social needs for which they seek health solutions. In a culturally heterogeneous country or one in which there is little continuity between the urban and rural experience, there may be even greater diversity of patient needs. The creation of a national health care system may limit the health care opportunities available through the strict consolidation of services and control of practitioners. The subsequent reduction of patient health care choices may affect negatively the patient's sense of having received proper care.

Developing countries such as Costa Rica need efficient, cost effective, and accessible health care services; these services are often best delivered by nationalized systems in which the financial burden of health care is equally shared by the individual, employer, and governmental agency. However, a system that is legislated without consideration of the first two points may produce more inefficiency and conflict than was initially expected. This risk, then, is of creating additional problems for the already strained and limited resources of the developing country. This risk must be evaluated and considered as part of a national health planning process which determines the best use of health care resources for population needs.

Developing countries are concerned about providing adequate health care for their populations; yet the problems these countries face are complex, and the conflicts are inherent in the very nature of our definition of development. Anthropology offers a methodology which can order this complexity and views the problems from the perspective of the patient in a cultural context. However, no matter what perspective the medical anthropologist prefers—the analysis of doctor-patient interaction, the description of health sectors, the study of the health seeking process, or the ethnography of health culture—he or she must also research the sociopolitical ideology and institutions that influence these other processes and conflict with otherwise culturally acceptable health behavior. The multilevel health behavior model enables the researcher to integrate the diverse levels of health care phenomena. The integration of the many social and cultural levels and processes of health behavior is the medical anthropology contribution to contemporary health care problems.

APPENDIX

AN OVERVIEW OF THE RESEARCH METHODOLOGY

The fieldsite was chosen after review of medical anthropological studies of complex health systems in Latin America (Foster 1962, 1969; Adams and Rubel 1967; Fabrega et al. 1967; Erasmus 1968; Fabrega and Metzger 1968; Press 1969, 1971, 1973; Richardson and Bode 1971; Teller 1972, 1973). The city in Latin America provides greater diversity of medical resources than any other culture system (Moore 1975); modern facilities are numerous and well-utilized, while "folk medical practitioners and treatments continue with vigor" (Press 1973). A broad spectrum of patients, services, and therapies is reflected in an urban medical system. The research problem required not only the diversity of the city, but also a culturally homogeneous population to minimize sociocultural variation. San José, the capital city of Costa Rica, offered this homogeneity as well as a cross-section of the entire hierarchy of political, economic, and administrative levels of the health care system.

The major portion of the research was undertaken in the San José outpatient clinics of four hospitals within the two principal Costa Rican health care delivery systems: Hospital Calderon Guardia and Hospital Mexico, of the Caja Costarricense de Seguro Social, and Hospital San Juan de Dios and psychiatric Hospital Manuel Antonio Chapui, of the Ministry of Public Health. The Caja Costarricense de Seguro Social is a semi-autonomous nationalized health, disability, and retirement program, which at the time of the study enrolled salaried employees and their families, some 60% of the total population (Caja Costarricense de Seguro Social 1974). The Ministry of Public Health is part of the executive branch of the central government which operates a lottery-supported system, providing free or low cost inpatient and outpatient care to those not covered by the Seguro Social. Additional field work was conducted with herbalists in the central market, pharmacists in their *boticas*, and with a range of paramedical practitioners in their offices and homes. Extensive ethnographic data were collected while living as a participant-observer in a transitional suburb of San José, where the researcher had informal contacts through everyday situations and personal interaction.

The methods employed varied according to the setting and sequence within the overall research design (Figure V). The initial phase of research was focused on medical administration interviews and observation of doctor-patient interaction in the consultation office. Between consultations, doctors, nurses, social workers, and other auxillary clinic personnel were interviewed with reference to their perceptions of patient behavior and clinic function. The second phase began after having established the pattern of consultation interaction; a structured interview covering patient perception of their illness and treatment was administered by a research assistant in the waiting room before and after the observed medical consultation. Finally, a sample of the interviewed patients were selected for a home visit, during which the researcher and her assistant conducted an open-ended family interview which emphasized personal and family health histories, genealogical and family network material, health utilization patterns, and general questions on values, preferences and health beliefs.

Observation of doctor-patient interaction was chosen as a means of most economically describing Costa Rican disease types, the variety of symptoms and their cultural expression, and doctor-patient interaction in terms of function and outcome. All observations of doctor-patient interaction and staff interviews were collected by the researcher—who was accompanied by a Costa Rican assistant[3] only in the initial meetings as a check on the researcher's language proficiency—thus eliminating the need for interviewer standardization. Consultations were recorded in notes taken in diary form and included relevant material on the situational context. The hospital outpatient general medicine clinics of the Public Health hospital, San Juan de Dios, and the Social Security hospital, Calderon Guardia, were selected to represent primary care services in San José. Two psychiatric clinics and one psychosomatic clinic were added to provide a perspective on secondary care.

The observed patient sample, distributed among the 7 clinics, was obtained by working alternate hours and days of the week with as many different doctors as possible; in this manner an

FIGURE V
Research Methods

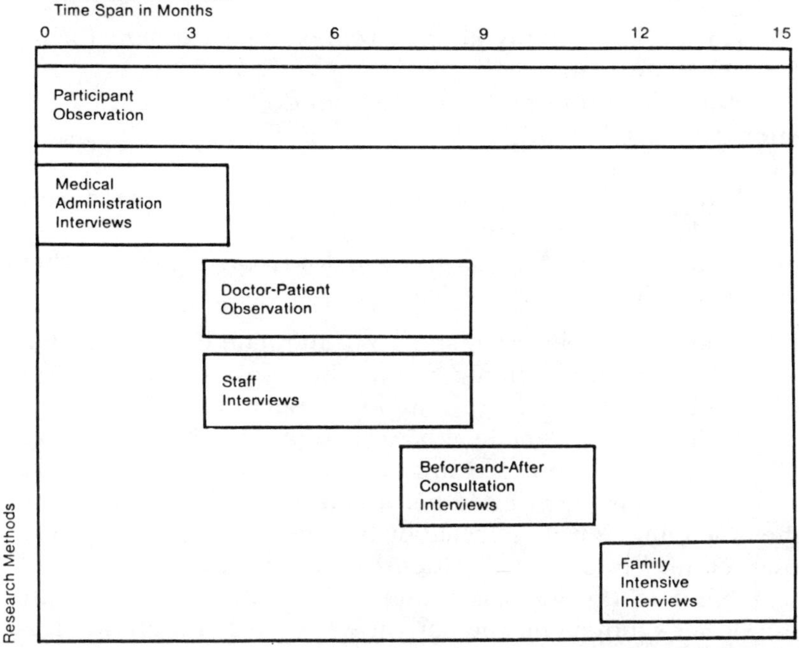

attempt was made to randomize patient attendance patterns. Approximately 12–20 patients were observed with each doctor depending on their case load. All patients who entered the office during the observation period were recorded to minimize selection bias. The 457 patient population constitutes a theoretical rather than a statistical sample.

The observation thus described yielded quantitative and qualitative data without intervention, but excluded patient perspective and comparison. Therefore, in the second phase of the research project, the observed patients were also interviewed before and after the consultation. A structured questionnaire elicited open-ended responses of patient expectations, concepts of disease causation and treatment, and satisfaction with the therapeutic encounter. The format was adopted from questions used in other cultural settings (Ordonez Plaja et al. 1968; Korsch and Negrete 1972) and structured to test hypotheses which developed through observations of doctor-patient interaction. The 117 before and after consultation interviews were collected by consecutively interviewing and observing consultations in each clinic setting.

While I was inside the medical consultation room, a research assistant asked patients the following questions:
(Before the consultation with the doctor)

1. What kind of problem do you have? Where did it come from?
2. Have you tried any kind of remedy or treatment for it? What have you tried?
3. What do you think the doctor can do for you?

(After the consultation)

4. How did it go? Why?
5. Did the doctor explain what you have? Did the doctor explain the treatment?
6. And now, what are you going to do? (return, go to another service, etc.)

The family sample was made up of the nine interviewed patients who agreed to a home visit by the research team and for whom there was also a consultation observation. They are a subsample of the larger health care study, in which a total of 457 patients were observed in a medical consultation with 117 of these patients interviewed before and after the consultation. The nine families were selected by the interviewer from the 117 observed and interviewed patients based on the receptivity of the patient to the idea of a home visit and whether, in the interviewer's judgment, the patient was verbal and knowledgeable. The families were chosen only to represent the seven clinics in the Public Health and Social Security institutions under study (at least one patient came from each clinic) and not because they were particularly representative of the clinic sample as a whole.

The intensive home interviews combined demographic factors, sociocultural variables, network analysis, and health histories of the entire household and provided intricate data on self-concept, cultural beliefs and attitudes, medical system utilization, and family organization. The home interview schedule (in English and Spanish) is available upon request from the author. The use of hypothetical illness situations tested ideal health behavior and lay referral system. (Friedson 1963; Weaver 1970). Open-ended questioning led to discussions of spiritual healing by Dr. Moreno Cañas (Vega Rodriguez 1958) and folk medicine preparation. These subjects were introduced by the patients during the interviews, which is suggestive of the importance of popular and folk medicine in the urban health system.

Participant observation in the communities where the researcher lived, in pharmacies, in paramedical and folk pracioners' offices and homes, and in the herbal section of the central market provided contextual background for the operating social and medical system. Discussions with social scientists and attendance at meetings of medical and pharmaceutical associations helped to clarify professional and academic points of view. The ethnographic task of learning the culture through interpersonal and social relationships supplemented the formal research process.

Analytic procedures were both quantitative and comparative. The 457 consultation observations were coded for 112 variables (including 65 possible symptom reports). The coding for doctor style and patient attitude followed a typology used by Ordonez Plaja, Cohen and Samora (1968) for doctor-patient interaction in Colombia. Patient requests and complaints were recorded from the 117 before and after consultation interviews according to a format suggested by Korsch and Negrete (1972) for doctor-patient communication in the United States. The majority of categories and scaling procedures, however, were derived from the empirical data using the naturally occurring variable groups and applying analytic descriptive labels. The body of interview materials were comparatively ordered by question, while participant observation records were organized by an outline of ethnographic topics modified for medical topics (Murdock et al. 1971). The data were then compared to theoretical questions and analytical models derived from the anthropological and health planning literature.

The data for the analysis of Dr. Moreno Cañas include documents published after his death, interviews with physicians who knew him, and interviews, observations, and references collected during the extensive study of health care in San José. Family members interviewed acknowledged healing by Dr. Moreno Cañas and reported their personal experiences. Medical journal articles, news accounts, and magazine editorials concerning Dr. Moreno Cañas' death, discovered during later research visits, expanded the information on his career and his development as a mythic figure. Materials on the Virgen de Los Angeles were collected both during interviews and during visits to the Basilica dedicated to the patron saint in Cartago.

NOTES

1. Bruce Newman, currently with INCAP of Guatemala, assisted me in the home interviews during which these questions were asked.

2. The interview schedule is available from the author upon request.

3. Norma Jiménez de Ramírez, of San José, Costa Rica, accompanied me to my initial medical consultations.

REFERENCES

Acuña, O. M.
n.d. The Family in Costa Rica. Heredia, Costa Rica: CESPO, Universidad Nacional de Costa Rica. Manuscript.

Adams, R.N.
1956 Cultural Components of Central America. American Anthropologist 58:881–907.

Adams, R.N. and A.J. Rubel
1967 Sickness and Social Relations. *In* Social Anthropology. Volume 6, Handbook of Middle American Indians. R. Wauchope, Ed. Austin: University of Texas Press.

Alford, R.R.
1975 Health Care Politics: Ideological and Interest Group Barriers to Reform. Chicago: University of Chicago Press.

Arrieta Q., Mons. V.M.
1960 La Patrona de Costa Rica. San José, Costa Rica: Imprenta Nacional, segunda edicion.

Asamblea Legislativa
1974 Código de Familia. Alcance No. 20 a La Gaceta No. 24. Diario Oficial. San José, Costa Rica. Martes 5 de Febrero.

Asuni, T.
1979 The Dilemma of Traditional Healing with Special Reference to Nigeria. Social Science and Medicine 13B:33–39.

Bell, J.P.
1971 Crisis in Costa Rica. The 1948 Revolution. Austin: University of Texas Press.

Bermúdez M.,V. and M. Gómez B.
1974 Panorama de Costa Rica, 1973: Aspectos Demográficos y Sociales. San José: CESPO.

Bertrand, W.E. and M. Micklin
1979 Attitudinal Classification of Health Manpower in Columbia: A Research on Urban/Rural Differences in Occupational Prestige. Social Science and Medicine 13A:235–240.

Bott, E.
1955 Urban Families: Conjugal Roles and Social Networks. Human Relations 8:345–384.
1957 Family and Social Networks, Roles, Norms and External Relationships of Ordinary Urban Families. New York: Free Press.

Bozzoli de Wille, M.E.
1971 No Creer Ni Dejar de Creer. Revista de Costa Rica 1:35–56, 2:67–84.

Bridgman, R.F.
1972 International Trends in Medical Care Organization and Research. *In* International Health Care. J. Fry and W.A.J. Farndale, Eds. Wallingford: Washington Square East.

Bursten, B.
1964 Family Dynamics and Illness Behavior. General Practitioner XXIX(5):142–145.

Bustamente Guerrero de Rivera, T.
1961 La Ciudad de San José. Ensayo Historico. Tesis de Licenciatura, Facultad de Ciencias y Letras, Universidad de Costa Rica.

Caja Costarricense de Seguro Social
1971 Reglamento del Seguro de Invalidez, Vejez y Muerte. Gaceta Oficial No. 142.
1972 Memoria 1972. San José, Costa Rica.
1974 Memoria 1973. San José, Costa Rica.

Caja Costarricense de Seguro Social, Sección de Relaciones Publicas
1973 Reglamento del Seguro de Enfermedad y Maternidad. San José, Costa Rica.

Caja Costarricense de Seguro Social, Departmento Actuarial Estadístico
1974 Informe Estadístico Trimestral 1974, 1er. trimestre. San José, Costa Rica.

Calvo, J. B.
1887 Apuntamientos Geográficos, Estadísticos é Históricos. San José: Imprenta Nacional.

Camacho C., E. M. and J. Alfaro M.
1977 La Seguridad Social en Costa Rica y La Llamada

"Deshumanización" de los Servicios Medicos. Revista Centroamericana de Ciencias de la Salud 8:75–96.

Casas, A. and H. Vargas

1980 The Health System in Costa Rica: Toward a National Health Service. Journal of Public Health Policy 1:258–279.

Chaves Camacho, J.

1969 Evolución Demografica de la Población de Costa Rica. Revista de la Universidad de Costa Rica 27:37–42.

Chrisman, N.J.

1977 The Health Seeking Process: An Approach to the Natural History of Illness. Culture, Medicine and Psychiatry 1(4):351–378.

Clark, M.

1970 Health in the Mexican American Culture. Berkeley and Los Angeles: University of California Press.

Colson, A.

1971 The Differential Use of Medical Resources in Developing Countries. Journal of Health and Social Behavior 12:226–237.

Cosminsky, S. and M. Scrimshaw

1980 Medical Pluralism on a Guatemalan Plantation. Social Science and Medicine 14B:267–278.

Croog, S.H.

1961 Ethnic Origins, Educational Levels and Responses to a Health Questionnaire. Human Organization 20:65–69.

Davis, M.S.

1968 Variation in Patients' Compliance with the Doctors' Advice: An Empirical Analysis of Patterns of Communication. American Journal of Public Health 58:274–288.

1971 Variation in Patients' Compliance with Doctors' Orders: Medical Practice and Doctor-Patient Interaction. Psychiatry in Medicine 2:31.

Debacher, D.E.

1979 Cognitive Models and Health Decision Making. Medical Anthropology 10(2):10–17.

de Miguel, J.

1977 Policies and Politics of the Health Reforms in Southern European Countries: A Sociological Critique. Social Science and Medicine 11:379–393.

de Mora, N.

1973 San José: Su Desarrallo, Su Titulo de Ciudad, Su

Rango de Capital de Costa Rica. Publicaciones de la Universidad de Costa Rica, Serie Misceláneas No. 154.

Denton, C.F.
1971 Patterns of Costa Rican Politics. Boston: Allyn and Bacon.

Departamento de Información Comercial
1982 Datos y Cifras de Costa Rica: Facts and Figures. San José, Costa Rica.

Diaz, M.N.
1970 Tonalá. Conservation, Responsibility, and Authority in a Mexican Town. Los Angeles and Berkeley: University of California Press.

Dobkin de Rios, M.
1981 Socio-characteristics of an Amazon Urban Healer's Clientele. Social Science and Medicine 15B:51–64.

Elling, R.H.
1978 Medical Systems as Changing Social Systems. Social Science and Medicine 12(2B):107–116.

El Seguro
1980 La Operación que Conmovió a Costa Rica: Dr. Moreno Cañas. Mayo/Junio, pp. 6–7.

Engelhardt, H.
1976 Ideology and Etiology. The Journal of Medicine and Philosophy 1:256–260.

Erasmus, C.J.
1968 An Anthropologist Looks at Technical Assistance. *In* Readings in Anthropology. M. Fried, Ed. New York: Thomas Y. Crowell.

Fabrega, H. and P.K. Manning
1979 Illness Episodes, Illness Severity and Treatment Options in a Pluralistic Setting. Social Science and Medicine 13B:41–51.

Fabrega, H. and D. Metzger
1968 Psychiatric Illness in a Small Ladino Community. Psychiatry 31:339–351.

Fabrega, H., A. Rubel and C.A. Wallace
1967 Working Class Mexican Psychiatric Outpatients. Archives of General Psychiatry 16:704–712.

Fabrega, H. and M. Zucker
1979 Components of Illness and Type of Medical Practitioner: A Comparative Study. Social Science and Medicine 13A:13–23.

Fallas, C.L.

1973 Mi Madrina. San José, Costa Rica: Editorial Costa Rica.

Farge, E.

1978 Medical Orientation Among a Mexican American Population: An Old and a New Model Reviewed. Social Science and Medicine 12:277–282.

Fendall, N.R.E.

1972 Medical Care in the Developing Nations. *In* International Health Care. J. Fry and W.A.J. Farndale, Eds., Wallingford: Washington Square East.

Ferguson, A.E.

1981 Commercial Pharmaceutical Medicine and Medicalization: A Case Study from El Salvador. Culture, Medicine and Psychiatry 5:105–134.

Field, M.G.

1973 The Concept of the Health System at the Macro-Sociological Level. Social Science and Medicine 7:763–785.

1980 The Health System and the Polity: A Contemporary American Dialectic. Social Science and Medicine 14A:397–441.

Finkler, K.

1980 Non-medical Treatments and Their Outcomes. Culture, Medicine and Psychiatry 4:271–310.

Foster, G.M.

1962 Traditional Cultures and the Impact of Technological Change. New York: Harper and Row.

1969 Applied Anthropology. Boston: Little, Brown.

1978 Medical Anthropology: Some Contrasts with Medical Sociology. *In* Health and the Human Condition. M.H. Logan and E.E. Hunt, Eds. North Scituate: Duxbury Press.

Fox, R.C.

1977 The Medicalization and Demedicalization of American Society. *In* Doing Better and Feeling Worse. J. H. Knowles, Ed. New York: W.W. Norton and Company.

Frankenberg, R.

1980 Medical Anthropology and Development: A Theoretical Perspective. Social Science and Medicine 14B: 197–207.

Freeman, B., et al.

1971 Gaps in Doctor-Patient Communication: Doctor-

Patient Interaction Analysis. Pediatric Research 5:298–311.

Friedson, E.

1960 Client Control and Medical Practice. American Journal of Sociology 65:374–382.

1963 Medical Care and the Public: Case Study of a Medical Group. Annals of the American Academy of Political and Social Science 346:57–66.

1970 Professional Dominance: The Social Structure of Medical Care. New York: Atherton.

1973 Prepaid Group Practice and the New Demanding Patient. Milbank Memorial Fund Quarterly 51:473–488.

Garrison, V.

1977 Doctor, *Espiritista* or Psychiatrist?: Health-Seeking Behavior in a Puerto Rican Neighborhood of New York City. Medical Anthropology 2:67–180.

Goffman, E.

1961 Asylums: Essays on the Social Situation of Mental Patients and Other Inmates. Chicago: Aldine.

Goldberg, E.M.

1958 Family Influences and Psychosomatic Illness: An Inquiry into the Social and Psychological Background of Duodenal Ulcer. London: Tavistock.

Good, C.M., J.M. Hunter, S. Katz and S. Katz

1979 The Interface of Dual Systems of Health Care in the Developing World: Toward Health Policy Initiatives in Africa. Social Science and Medicine 13D:141–154.

Gray, L.C.

1980 Consumer Satisfaction with Physician Provided Services: A Panel Study. Social Science and Medicine 14A:65–73.

Green, E. C.

1980 Roles for African Traditional Healers in Mental Health Care. Medical Anthropology 4(4):489–522.

Gutierrez Saenz, R.

1971 Distribución Geográfica, Institucional y por Actividad de Los Médicos en Costa Rica. Ciudad Universitaria Costa Rica, Facultad de Medicina.

Harrison, P.

1981 Success Story. World Health, February–March, pp. 14–19.

Heath, D.B.

1974 Introduction to Social Groupings and Authority. *In*

Contemporary Cultures and Societies of Latin America. D.B. Heath, Ed., New York: Random House.

Heggenhougen, H.K.

1980 The Utilization of Traditional Medicine: A Malaysian Example. Social Science and Medicine 14B:39–44.

Hill, C.E.

1973 Convitiendose en Campesinos: Los Boruca de Costa Rica. America Indígena 33(2):447–456.

Hollingshead, A.B. and F.C. Redlich

1958 Social Class and Mental Illness. New York: John Wiley and Sons.

Idler, E.L.

1979 Definitions of Health and Illness and Medical Sociology. Social Science and Medicine 13A:723–731.

Igun, U.A.

1979 Stages in Health-Seeking: A Descriptive Model. Social Science and Medicine 13A(4):445–456.

Illich, I.

1976 Medical Nemesis: The Expropriation of Health. New York: Pantheon Books.

Jackson, D. and I. Yalom

1966 Family Research on the Problem of Ulcerative Colitis. Archives of General Psychiatry 15:410–418.

James, P.

1959 Latin America. New York: Odyssey.

Janzen, J.M.

1978 The Comparative Study of Medical Systems as Changing Social Systems. Social Science and Medicine 12(2B):121–130.

Jaramillo Antillón, J.

1983 Los Problemas de la Salud en Costa Rica. Políticas y Estrategies. San José, Costa Rica: Litografía Ambar.

Kane, T.T.

1979 World Fertility Survey Update: Costa Rica. Intercom, March, p. 14.

Kasl, S.V. and S. Cobb

1966 Health Behavior, Illness Behavior and Sick Role Behavior. Archives of Environmental Health 12:246–266.

Kassebaum, G.G. and B. Baumann

1965 Diversities in Conceptions of Health and Physical Fitness. Journal of Health and Human Behavior 6:16–27.

Kleinman, A.

1978 Concepts and a Model for the Comparison of Medical Systems as Cultural Systems. Social Science and Medicine 12(2B):85–94.

1980 Patients and Healers in the Context of Culture. Berkeley: University of California.

Kleinman, A. and L.H. Sung

1979 Why Do Indigenous Practitioners Successfully Heal? Social Science and Medicine 13B:7–26.

Korsch, B. et al.

1968 Gaps in Doctor-Patient Communication: Doctor-Patient Interaction and Patient Satisfaction. Pediatrics 42:855–871.

Korsch, B.M. and V.F. Negrete

1972 Doctor-Patient Communication. Scientific American 227:66–75.

Kurella, S.

1979 The Social Needs of Patients and Their Satisfaction with Medical Care: A Survey of Medical Inpatients in the Country Hospitals of the German Democratic Republic. Social Science and Medicine 13A:737.

La Nación

1982 Costa Rica Médicos se Acercan a Las Seis Semanas en Huelga. 4–10 de Junio, p. 3.

La Republica

1973 News Report. San José, Costa Rica, p. 12.

Larsen, D.E. and I. Rootman

1976 Physician Role Performance and Patient Satisfaction. Social Science and Medicine 10:29–32.

Lasker, J.N.

1977 The Role of Health Services in Colonial Rule: The Case of the Ivory Coast. Culture, Medicine and Psychiatry 1(3):277–297.

Lebow, J.L.

1974 Consumer Assessments of the Quality of Medical Care. Medical Care 12:328.

Leeds, A.

1968 The Anthropology of Cities: Some Methodological Issues. *In* Urban Anthropology: Research Perspectives and Strategies. E.M. Eddy, Ed. Southern Anthropological Society Proceedings, No. 2. Athens: University of Georgia.

Leslie, C., Ed.

1976 Asian Medical Systems. Berkeley: University of California Press.

Locker, D. and D. Dunt

1978 Theoretical and Methodological Issues in Sociological Studies of Consumer Satisfaction with Medical Care. Social Science and Medicine 12:283–292.

Low, S.M.

1977 Costa Rican Family Structure. *In* First Child and Family Formation. W. Miller and L. Newman, Eds., Chapel Hill: Population Center.

1981 The Meaning of *Nervios*: A Sociocultural Analysis of Symptom Presentation in San José, Costa Rica. Culture, Medicine and Psychiatry 3:1–26.

1982 Dr. Moreno Cañas: A Symbolic Bridge to the Demedicalization of Healing. Social Science and Medicine 16:527–531.

Mabry, J.H.

1964 Medicine and the Family. Journal of Marriage and the Family, May: 160–165.

Maclean, C.M.U.

1966 Hospitals or Healers? An Attitude Survey in Ibadan. Human Organization 25:131–139.

MacLeod, M.J.

1973 Spanish Central America: A Socioeconomic History 1520–1720. Berkeley: University of California Press.

Mburu, F.M.

1981 Implications of the Ideology and Implementation of Health Policy in a Developing Country. Social Science and Medicine 15A:17–24.

Mechanic, D.

1963 Religion, Religiosity and Illness Behavior: The Special Case of the Jews. Human Organization 22:202–208.

1966 Response Factors in Illness: The Study of Illness Behavior. Social Psychiatry 1:11–20.

1976 The Growth of Bureaucratic Medicine: An Inquiry into the Dynamics of Patient Behavior and the Organization of Medical Care. New York: John Wiley.

Ministerio de Economía, Industria y Comercio

1970 Anuario Comercio Exterior. San José, Costa Rica.

Ministerio de Economía, Industria y Comerico, Dirección General de Estadística y Censos

1972 Estadística Vital. San José, Costa Rica.

1974 Censo de Poblacion 1973. Tomo 1. San José, Costa Rica.

Ministerio de Salubridad Publica
1973 Projecto de Ley Organica del Ministerio de Salubridad Publica. San José, Costa Rica.

Ministerio de Salud
1974 Memoria Anual 1973. San José, Costa Rica.
1975 Memoria Anual 1974. San José, Costa Rica.

Ministerio de Salud, Departamento de Estadística
1974 Informaciones Estadísticas Anuario de 1973. Sistema Hospicio Nacional, Unidades Sanitarias y Otras Progamas de Salud. San José, Costa Rica.

Minuchin, S., B.L. Rosman and L. Baker
1978 Psychosomatic Families: Anorexia Nervosa in Context. Cambridge: Harvard University Press.

Monge Alfaro, C.
1974 Historia de Costa Rica. San José: Trejos Hermanos.

Moore, K.
1975 The City as Context: Context as Process. Urban Anthropology 4(1):017–026.

Murdock, G.P., and C.S. Ford, A.E. Hudson, R. Kennedy, L.W. Simmons and J.W.M. Whiting
1971 Outline of Cultural Materials. 4th edition. New Haven: Human Relations Area Files.

Murphy, J.M.
1976 Psychiatric Labeling in Cross-Cultural Perspective. Science 191:1019–1025.

Myerhoff, B. and W.R. Larsen
1965 The Doctor as Culture Hero: The Routinization of Charisma. Human Organization 24:188–191.

Nathanson C.A.
1977 Sex, Illness and Medical Care: A Review of Data, Theory and Method. Social Science and Medicine 11:13–25.

Navarro, V.
1978 Class Struggle, the State and Medicine: An Historical and Contemporary Analysis of the Medical Sector in Great Britain. New York: Prodist.

Newman, M.T. and B. Newman
1974 Reduction of Population Growth: The Costa Rican Case. Paper presented at the American Anthropological Association Meetings, Mexico City. November.

Ness, R.C.
1980 The Impact of Indigenous Healing Activity: An Empirical Study of Two Fundamentalist Churches. Social Science and Medicine 14B:167–180.

Nichter, M.

1978 Patterns of Resort in the Use of Therapy Systems and Their Significance for Health Planning in South Asia. Medical Anthropology 2(2):29–58.

1980 The Layperson's Perception of Medicine as Perspective into the Utilization of Multiple Therapy Systems in the Indian Context. Social Science and Medicine 14B:225–233.

Ordonez Plaja, A., L.M. Cohen and J. Samora

1968 Communication Between Physicians and Patients in Outpatient Clinics. Milbank Memorial Fund Quarterly 46:161–213.

Osterweis, M., P.J. Bush and A.E. Zuckerman.

1979 Family Context as a Predictor of Individual Medicine Use. Social Science and Medicine 13A:287–291.

Parsons, T.

1958 Definitions of Health and Illness in the Light of American Values and Social Structure. *In* Patients, Physicians and Illness. E. Jaco Ed. Glencoe: Free Press.

Parsons, T. and R. Fox.

1952 Illness, Therapy and the Modern Urban American Family. Journal of Social Issues 8(4):31–55.

Paul, B.D., Ed.

1955 Health, Culture and Community. New York: Russell Sage.

Pearce, T.O.

1980 Political and Economic Changes in Nigeria and the Organization of Medical Care. Social Science and Medicine 14B:91–98.

Peattie, L.R.

1970 The View from the Barrio. Ann Arbor: University of Michigan Press.

Pellegrino, E.D.

1963 Medicine, History and the Idea of Man. Annals of the American Academy of Political and Social Sciences 346:9–20.

Press, I.

1969 Urban Illness: Physicians, Curers and Dual Use in Bogota. Journal of Health and Social Behavior 10:209–17.

1971 The Urban Curandero. American Anthropologist 73(3):741–56.

1973 Bureaucracy Versus Folk Medicine: Implication from Seville, Spain. Urban Anthropology 2(2):232–47.

1980 Problems in the Definition and Classification of Medical Systems. Social Science and Medicine 14B:45–58.

Richardson, M. and B. Bode

1971 Popular Medicine in Puntarenas, Costa Rica: Urban and Societal Features. Publication 24:249–275. Middle American Research Institute, Tulane University.

Rodríguez Vega, E.

1953 Apuntes Para una Sociología Costarricense. San José, Costa Rica: Sección Tesis de Grado y Ensayos, No. 4.

Romannucci Schwartz, L.

1969 The Hierarchy of Resort in Curative Practices: The Admiralty Islands, Melanesia. Journal of Health and Social Behavior 10:201–209.

Rosenberg, M.B.

1981 Social Reform in Costa Rica: Social Security and the Presidency of Rafael Angel Calderon. Hispanic American Historical Review 61:278–296.

Rubel, A.J.

1964 The Epidemiology of a Folk Illness: "Susto" in Hispanic America. Ethnology 3:268–283.

1966 Across the Tracks. Austin: University of Texas.

Sancho, M.

1935 Suiza Centro Americana. San José: Talleres Tipograficos "La Tribuna".

Schapiro, M.H.

1962 Apuntes Sobre la Evolución Médica en Costa Rica 1780–1930. Revista Médica de Costa Rica 29:489–499, 30:33–39.

Schuster, L.

1981 Riches to Rags. The Wall Street Journal CXCVIII: 85, October 29, pp.1, 12.

Segall, A.

1976 The Sick Role Concept: Understanding Illness Behavior. Journal of Health and Social Behavior 17:163–170.

Segovia, R.

1951 Estudio de la Clase Media en Costa Rica. *En* Materiales para el Estudio de la Clase Media en la America Latina V. Union Panamericana, Washington, D.C.

Seligson, M.A.

1974 Agrarian Capitalism and the Transformation of Peasant Society: Coffee in Costa Rica. Unpublished manuscript. Department of Government, University of Arizona.

1980 Peasants of Costa Rica and the Development of Agrarian Capitalism. Madison: University of Wisconsin Press.

Solis Zeledon, R., R. Ferrer de Beck, and F. Marin Ch.

1969 Deliminación de la Region Metropolitana de San José. San José, Costa Rica: Instituto Nacional de Vivenda y Urbanismo.

Stephens, J.L.

1949 Incidents of Travel in Central America, Chiapas and Yucatan. Vol. I. New Brunswick: Rutgers University.

Stone, S.

1969 Los Cafetaleros: Un Estudio de los Grandes Caficultores de Costa Rica. Revista de Ciencias Jurídicas. Universidad de Costa Rica, No. 13.

1974 Aspects of Power Distribution in Costa Rica. *In* Contemporary Cultures and Societies of Latin America. D.B. Heath, Ed. New York: Random House.

Suchman, E.A.

1964 Sociomedical Variations Among Ethnic Groups. American Journal of Sociology 70:319–331.

Svarstad, B.L.

1976 Physician-Patient Communication and Patient Conformity with Medical Advice. *In* The Growth of Bureaucratic Medicine. D. Mechanic, Ed. New York: John Wiley.

Teller, C.H.

1972 Internal Migration, Socioeconomic Status and Health: Access to Medical Care in a Honduran City. Latin American Studies Program. Dissertation Series no. 41, Cornell University.

1973 Access to Medical Care of Migrants in a Honduran City. Journal of Health and Social Behavior 14:214–266.

Thein, T.M.

1974 Contraception in Costa Rica: A Sociocultural Study of Three Communities. Ph.D. dissertation. Graduate School of Arts and Sciences, Columbia University.

Titchener, J.L., J. Riskin and R. Emerson

1960 The Family in Psychosomatic Process. Psychosomatic Medicine 22 (2):127–42.

Townsend, J.M. and C.L. Carbone

1980 Menopausal Syndrome: Illness or Social Role, a

Transcultural Analysis. Culture, Medicine and Psychiatry 4:229–248.

Turner, R.H.

1970 Family Interaction. New York: John Wiley.

Ugalde, A.

1978 Health Decision Making in Developing Nations: A Comparative Analysis of Colombia and Iran. Social Science and Medicine 12:1–7.

1980 Physicians' Control of the Health Sector. Professional Values and Economic Interests: Findings from the Honduran Health System. Social Science and Medicine 14A:435–444.

Unschuld, P.U.

1979 Comparative Systems of Health Care. Social Science and Medicine 13A(5):523–528.

Vayda, A.P.

1974 Warfare in Ecological Perspective. Annual Review of Ecology and Systematics 5:183–193.

Vega Rodriguez, J.

1958 Vida, Pasión y Muerte del Dr. Ricardo Moreno Cañas. *In* Sociedad Cuban de Historia. Carlos de la Torre y Huerta, Ed. Habana: Natural "Felipe Poey," No. 3.

Verbrugge, L.M.

1978 Sex and Gender in Health and Medicine. Social Science and Medicine 12:329–333.

Von Bulow, T.

1974 Apuntes para la Historia de la Medicina en Costa Rica durante la Colonia. Revista de Costa Rica 5:115–140.

Waitzkin, H.

1979 Medicine, Superstructure and Micropolitics. Social Science and Medicine 13A:601–609.

Weaver, T.

1970 Use of Hypothetical Situations in a Study of Spanish American Illness Referral Systems. Human Organization 29(2):140–154.

Weidman, H.

1979 The Transcultural View: Prerequisite to Interethnic (Intercultural) Communication in Medicine. Social Science and Medicine 13B:85–87.

West, R.C. and J.P. Augelli

1966 Middle America: Its Land and People. Englewood Cliffs: Prentice-Hall.

Willems, E.

1968 Urban Classes and Acculturation in Latin America. *In* Urban Anthropology. E.M. Eddy, Ed. Southern Anthropological Proceedings, No. 2

Woolley, F.R.,L. Kane, C.C. Hughes and D.D. Wright

1978 Research note: The Effects of Doctor-Patient Communication on Satisfaction and Outcome of Care. Social Science and Medicine 12:123–128.

Wolf, E. and E.C. Hansen

1972 The Human Condition in Latin America. New York: Oxford.

Wolff, B.B. and S. Langley

1968 Cultural Factors and Pain Response: A Review. American Anthropologist 70:494–501.

Woods, C.M.

1977 Alternative Curing Strategies in a Changing Medical Situation. Medical Anthropology 3:26–54.

Young, A.

1976 Some Implications for Medical Beliefs and Practice for Social Anthropology. American Anthropologist 78:5–24.

Young, J.C.

1980 A Model of Illness Treatment in a Tarascan Town. American Ethnologist 7(1):106–131.

1981 Medical Choice in a Mexican Village. New Brunswick: Rutgers University Press.

Zborowski, M.

1952 Cultural Components in Responses to Pain. Journal of Social Issues 8:16–30.

Zola, I.K.

1966 Culture and Symptoms: An Analysis of Patients' Presenting Complaints. American Sociological Review 31:615–630.

1973 Pathways to the Doctor—From Person to Patient. Social Science and Medicine 7:677–589.

INDEX